Multiple Chemical Sensitivity
M.C.S.

"Understand the Essentials"

Marc Sachot

Print on Demand
Legal Deposit: August 2024
ISBN: 978-2-9589939-4-8

National Library of France

Price (including VAT): $17

Preface

Welcome to these pages that aim to shed light on a complex and often misunderstood subject: Multiple Chemical Sensitivity (MCS) or Idiopathic Environmental Intolerance (IEI). In this preface, I wish to share with you my personal journey and what led me to write this book, particularly for healthcare professionals.

My experience with MCS began in 2012, while I was working as a production engineer in a plastics company. Following exposure to dust containing nickel and other toxic substances at my workplace, I faced a series of inexplicable and debilitating symptoms. From persistent headaches and recurrent nausea to skin rashes, memory loss, and overwhelming chronic fatigue, each day became a battle against my own environment. In search of answers, I discovered the complex world of chemical sensitivities and environmental intolerances, where seemingly insignificant odors and contact with certain materials could trigger devastating reactions.

This personal struggle drove me to dive deep into research, to explore the underlying mechanisms of MCS, and to understand the challenges faced by those affected by this condition. This book is the result of that exploration and was developed from books published by renowned doctors as well as medical publications. It aims to demystify MCS, provide practical advice for daily management, and, most importantly, offer a message of hope to those who often feel isolated in their struggle.

Through these pages, we will explore the origins of MCS, the symptoms that characterize it, the challenges of diagnosis, treatment options, and adaptation strategies. We will also hear from medical experts and provide practical advice for navigating a world that can sometimes seem hostile. My goal is for this book to become a valuable resource for healthcare professionals, helping them better understand this complex condition, recognize its manifestations, and offer appropriate support to their patients.

Healthcare professionals play a crucial role in the diagnosis and management of MCS. By better understanding this condition, they can not only offer more effective care but also help reduce the stigma often associated with MCS. I am convinced that this book will provide new insights and practical tools to improve the care of patients with MCS.

However, it is essential to emphasize that this book is informative and that I cannot be held responsible for the application of specific advice. It is imperative that everyone consults their doctor for personalized advice tailored to their particular medical situation.

Thank you for joining me in this exploration. Together, we can break down the barriers of stigma, promote compassion, and advance the cause of those living with MCS.

With all my support,

Marc

Table of contents

Chapter 1: What is chemical sensitivity?

Chapter 2: A day in the life

Chapter 3: Health impact

Chapter 4: Diagnosing chemical sensitivity

Chapter 5: Living with restrictions

Chapter 6: Treatments for a better quality of life

Theron Grant Randolph

(July 7, 1906 – September 29, 1995)

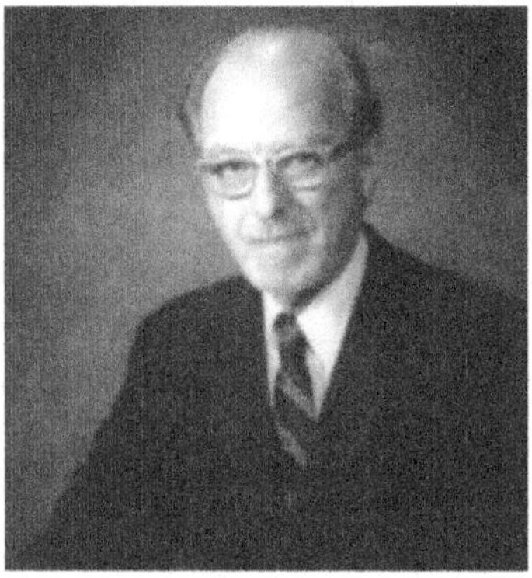

An American physician and allergist recognized as the "Father of Clinical Ecology." He studied food allergies and chemical sensitivities, challenging the medical views of his time. His research contributed to the recognition of chemical sensitivities and the founding of environmental medicine.

Chapter 1
What is chemical sensitivity?

1.1 Definition and terminology, history and discovery

Definition and terminology:

Chemical sensitivity, often referred to as Multiple Chemical Sensitivity (MCS), is a medical condition in which an individual develops symptoms after exposure to low levels of chemicals commonly found in the environment. These chemicals include solvents, cleaning products, perfumes, pesticides, plastics, and building materials, among others. Symptoms are highly varied and can include headaches, dizziness, respiratory difficulties, cognitive issues, and skin problems.

The term "Multiple Chemical Sensitivity" (MCS) was first proposed by Dr. Theron Randolph (an American physician, allergist, and researcher) in the 1950s. He observed that some of his patients experienced physical reactions to low levels of common chemicals, and he suggested that these reactions might be due to an increased sensitivity to these substances. Since then, other terms have been used to describe this phenomenon, such as "Idiopathic Environmental Intolerance" (IEI) and "Toxicant-Induced Loss of Tolerance" (TILT).

History and discovery:

The history of chemical sensitivity dates back several decades. Here are some key points in its development and recognition:

- 1950 - 1960: The first descriptions of adverse reactions to low-level chemical exposures were reported by some doctors and scientists. Dr. Theron Randolph, an allergist and immunologist, was one of the pioneers in this field. He observed reactions in patients exposed to chemicals in both domestic and professional environments.

- 1970: Dr. William J. Rea, a thoracic surgeon and environmentalist, continued Dr. Randolph's work by founding the Environmental Health Center-Dallas. He contributed to advancing the understanding of MCS (Multiple Chemical Sensitivity) by examining the effects of chemical exposures on human health.

- 1980: The term "Multiple Chemical Sensitivity" was popularized by Dr. Theron Randolph. His work helped define and identify the specific symptoms of MCS, such as headaches, fatigue, respiratory issues, and neurological symptoms, often in response to low-level chemical exposures.

- 1990: Research and debate on MCS intensified. Dr. Claudia Miller, a professor of environmental medicine at the University of Texas, introduced the concept of Idiopathic Environmental Intolerance (IEI). Discussions often divided those who viewed MCS as a psychosomatic condition from those who saw it as a genuine physical pathology.

- 2000 and beyond: Research has intensified to understand the underlying mechanisms of MCS. Dr. Martin Pall, a biochemist, proposed a theory suggesting that MCS might be related to a biochemical cycle of oxidative stress and inflammatory response. Despite these advancements, there is still no universal consensus on the exact causes and standardized diagnostic criteria.

Chemical sensitivity is a complex and controversial area of environmental medicine. While many individuals report disabling symptoms associated with exposure to low levels of chemicals, recognition and understanding of this condition vary widely among healthcare professionals. Ongoing research is crucial to clarify the underlying mechanisms and develop effective management strategies for those affected.

1.2 Common symptoms

The symptoms of Multiple Chemical Sensitivity are varied and can affect different systems of the body. They are often triggered by exposure to low levels of common chemicals in the environment, and their severity varies from person to person. Here is a detailed description of common symptoms associated with MCS:

1. Respiratory symptoms:

Respiratory symptoms include difficulty breathing (shortness of breath), asthma-like symptoms such as wheezing and persistent cough, as well as issues with nasal congestion, runny nose, and sinusitis.

2. Neurological and cognitive symptoms:

Neurological symptoms include headaches, including migraines, sensations of dizziness or lightheadedness, cognitive disorders such as mental confusion, short-term memory problems, and difficulty concentrating. Additionally, persistent extreme fatigue is often present.

3. Gastrointestinal symptoms:

Gastrointestinal symptoms include nausea and vomiting after chemical exposure, abdominal pain with possible cramping, as well as gastrointestinal disorders such as diarrhea or constipation.

4. Musculoskeletal symptoms:

Individuals frequently experience muscle and joint pain, often described as generalized discomfort. Additionally, some may also experience a sensation of muscle weakness.

5. Dermatological symptoms:

Individuals may develop rashes, itching, and redness after exposure, as well as hives, a form of allergic skin reaction.

6.Cardiac symptoms:

Symptoms of palpitations, characterized by irregular or rapid heartbeats, as well as chest pain similar to that of angina, are frequently experienced by individuals.

7. Psychological and emotional symptoms:

Anxiety and depressive disorders are frequently reported in individuals with MCS. Symptoms also include mood swings, increased irritability, and rapid changes in mood, which are attributed to the condition.

Symptoms are varied and affect almost all body systems. Their heterogeneous and often subjective presentation makes diagnosis difficult, and patients face challenges in obtaining recognition and appropriate treatment. Healthcare professionals need to be attentive to these diverse manifestations to provide appropriate support and care for those affected by MCS. Ongoing research is essential to better understand these reactions and develop effective management strategies.

1.3 Types of chemical sensitivities

MCS encompasses various reactions to chemicals present in the environment. Types of chemical sensitivities are classified based on the specific substances or categories of chemicals that trigger symptoms. Here is a detailed description of the main types of chemical sensitivities:

1.Sensitivity to organic solvents:

Hydrocarbons such as benzene, toluene, and xylene, commonly used in paints, varnishes, and adhesives, trigger reactions in individuals sensitive to these products. Similarly, substances such as acetone, used in nail polish removers, and ethanol, present in disinfectants and some beverages, are also triggers. Additionally, ethers and esters used in perfumes, cleaning products, and industrial applications can cause symptoms in certain sensitive individuals.

2. Sensitivity to pesticides:

Insecticides, such as organophosphates and carbamates used to kill insects, as well as herbicides like glyphosate used to eliminate weeds, are likely to trigger reactions in individuals sensitive to chemicals. Additionally, fungicides, toxic substances used to control fungi and mold, also pose problems for these individuals.

3. Sensitivity to cleaning products:

Household cleaning products, containing substances such as chlorine, ammonia, and phenols, trigger reactions in individuals sensitive to chemicals. Similarly, chemical compounds found in laundry detergents, fabric softeners, and all-purpose cleaners are also likely to cause symptoms in these individuals.

4. Sensitivity to personal care products:

Fragrances present in perfumes, lotions, and shampoos trigger reactions in individuals sensitive to chemicals. Additionally, preservatives such as parabens and sulfates, as well as other additives commonly used in personal care products, act as triggers. Artificial colorants and texture agents found in cosmetics can also provoke reactions in some people sensitive to chemicals.

5. Sensitivity to building materials:

Volatile organic compounds (VOCs) found in paints, varnishes, and coatings are triggers for chemical sensitivity. Similarly, adhesives, sealants, and glues used in various contexts can provoke symptoms. Additionally, certain building materials such as particle board, carpets, and insulation can release chemicals that trigger reactions in sensitive individuals.

6. Sensitivity to food products and additives:

Food preservatives such as sulfites and nitrites, commonly used to extend the shelf life of foods, have the potential to trigger reactions in sensitive individuals. Similarly, artificial food colorants found in many processed foods are sometimes associated with undesirable reactions. Additionally, artificial flavors used to enhance the taste of foods can be problematic for those sensitive to chemicals.

Chemical sensitivities are varied and include reactions to a wide range of chemicals present in our daily environment. Recognizing specific types of chemical sensitivities is essential for diagnosing and managing symptoms in individuals. A better understanding of specific triggers allows for more effective avoidance and treatment strategies, thus improving quality of life. Ongoing research is crucial to deepen our understanding of these sensitivities and to develop tailored management approaches.

1.4 Risk factors and possible causes

MCS is a complex condition with its exact causes remaining poorly understood. However, several risk factors and possible causes have been identified. These include genetic factors, environmental exposures, medical history, and psychological aspects. Here is a detailed description of the risk factors and possible causes of MCS:

1. Risk factors:

   1. Prolonged exposure to chemicals:

      - *Work environment:* Individuals working in industries where they are regularly exposed to chemicals, such as painters, hairstylists, agricultural workers, and factory workers, have an increased risk of developing MCS.

      - *Home environment:* Continuous exposure to household toxic products such as cleaning agents, perfumes, and personal care products also increases the risk.

   2. Genetic predisposition:

      - *Family history:* Individuals with family members who have MCS or other disorders related to chemical exposure are more likely to develop MCS themselves.

      - *Genetic variations:* Specific genetic variations may make certain individuals more vulnerable to the effects of environmental chemicals.

3. Preexisting medical conditions:

- *Allergies and asthma:* Individuals with a history of allergies or asthma are more likely to develop chemical sensitivities.

- *Autoimmune disorders:* Individuals with autoimmune disorders also have an increased risk.

4. Stress and psychological factors:

- *Chronic stress:* High levels of chronic stress can weaken the immune system and make a person more vulnerable to chemical sensitivities.

- *Anxiety and depression:* Individuals suffering from anxiety or depressive disorders may be more sensitive to the effects of chemicals.

2. Possible causes:

1. Toxic load hypothesis:

The toxic load hypothesis suggests that chemical sensitivity might result from a gradual accumulation of toxins in the body due to prolonged and repeated exposure to low levels of chemicals. Pollutants from various sources, such as cleaning products, pesticides, and solvents, accumulate in the body, and the body becomes unable to effectively detoxify these substances, leading to a toxic overload. This accumulation causes multisystemic symptoms, affecting various body systems, including the respiratory system, nervous system, and digestive system.

2. Immune system dysfunction:

Some theories suggest that MCS may be due to immune system dysfunction, where the immune system reacts excessively or inappropriately to environmental chemicals. Key elements of this hypothesis include abnormal immune responses, where the immune system reacts disproportionately to chemicals, and autoimmunity, where the immune system attacks the body's own tissues in response to chemical exposures. Additionally, these abnormal reactions can lead to chronic systemic inflammation, contributing to MCS symptoms.

3. Central nervous system hypersensitivity:

The central sensitization theory suggests that chemical sensitivity may be linked to hypersensitivity of the central nervous system, where the brain and spinal cord amplify pain and distress signals in response to chemical exposures. Key points of this hypothesis include central sensitization, where the nervous system amplifies pain signals, and neurological dysfunction, involving chemical imbalances and alterations in neurotransmitters that increase sensitivity to chemicals. This hypersensitivity may explain the neurological and cognitive symptoms frequently observed in affected individuals.

4. Systemic inflammation:

The inflammatory response theory proposes that exposure to chemicals triggers inflammatory reactions throughout the body, contributing to the various symptoms observed in individuals with MCS. Key aspects include systemic inflammatory reactions induced by environmental chemicals, the release of proinflammatory cytokines[1] and other inflammatory mediators that contribute to MCS symptoms, and chronic inflammation that may lead to tissue damage and exacerbate symptoms.

5. Oxidative imbalance:

The oxidative stress theory suggests that chemical sensitivity is linked to an imbalance between free radicals and antioxidants in the body, caused by chemical exposure. Key aspects of this hypothesis include excessive production of free radicals due to chemical exposure, oxidative imbalance where the excess of free radicals[2] compared to antioxidants leads to cellular damage, and systemic effects of oxidative stress that impact various body systems, resulting in multisystemic symptoms.

6. Psychosocial factors:

Some research suggests that psychosocial factors, such as stress, anxiety, and negative expectations regarding chemical exposure, can play a role in the development and exacerbation of chemical sensitivity symptoms. Key elements of this theory include chronic stress and anxiety disorders, which increase susceptibility to chemical sensitivities; the nocebo effect, where negative expectations amplify symptoms; and psychosomatic

---

1 Cytokines, immune system proteins, regulate immune and inflammatory responses. In MCS, they may be released in response to chemicals, contributing to inflammation and symptoms.

2 Free radicals are unstable molecules that can damage cells. They are naturally produced in the body, but their accumulation, often due to environmental exposures, can contribute to diseases.

interactions, where psychological factors interact with physiological factors to worsen symptoms.

Multiple chemical sensitivity is a multifactorial condition with its exact causes still unknown. Several theories explain chemical sensitivity, offering different perspectives on its mechanisms. MCS may be a multifactorial condition involving interactions between genetic, immunological, neurological, inflammatory, oxidative, and psychosocial factors. Ongoing research is essential to clarify these mechanisms and develop effective treatments.

1.5 Diagnostic challenges

Diagnosing MCS presents numerous challenges due to the complexity and subjective nature of the symptoms, as well as the lack of consensus within the medical community. Here is a detailed exploration of the main challenges in diagnosing the condition:

1. Symptom variability:

Symptoms vary significantly from person to person, affecting various body systems such as the respiratory, nervous, gastrointestinal, and skin systems, among others. This diversity makes it challenging to establish a consistent clinical picture. Additionally, symptoms fluctuate in intensity and frequency, complicating the direct correlation between chemical exposure and clinical manifestations.

2. Lack of objective biomarkers:

There is currently no specific laboratory test to diagnose MCS, making it difficult to base the diagnosis on objective evidence. Additionally, precisely quantifying exposure to low levels of environmental chemicals and establishing a clear link to specific symptoms is complex and often imprecise.

3. Psychosocial factors:

Symptoms are influenced by psychological factors such as stress, anxiety, and negative expectations, creating a complex interaction between the physical and psychological aspects of the condition. Additionally, MCS is sometimes perceived as a psychosomatic condition, leading to stigma for patients and skepticism from some healthcare professionals.

4. Differential diagnosis:

Symptoms are likely to resemble those of other medical conditions such as asthma, allergies, fibromyalgia, chronic fatigue syndrome, and other pathologies, complicating the differential diagnosis process. Additionally, an accurate diagnosis often requires the careful exclusion of other potential causes of the symptoms, making the process lengthy and complex for both healthcare professionals and patients.

5. Lack of consensus and diagnostic criteria:

There is no universal consensus on the diagnostic criteria for multiple chemical sensitivity syndrome, leading to variations in how the diagnosis is made by different practitioners and institutions. Additionally, the methods and evaluation protocols vary significantly, resulting in inconsistent diagnoses and increased difficulty for patients in obtaining appropriate medical recognition of their condition.

6. Problems related to self-diagnosis and public information:

Many patients turn to self-diagnosis due to the lack of medical recognition, leading to errors and inappropriate self-treatments. Additionally, the spread of unverified or incorrect information on the internet and in the media influences patients' perceptions and complicates clinical diagnosis.

Diagnosing chemical sensitivity is a complex challenge due to symptom variability, the absence of objective biomarkers, psychosocial factors, difficult differential diagnosis, lack of consensus on diagnostic criteria, and issues related to self-diagnosis. A collaborative approach among patients, clinicians, and researchers is crucial to improve the recognition, understanding, and management of MCS.

1.6 Prevalence and epidemiological data

The prevalence of MCS and associated epidemiological data are essential for understanding the impact of this condition on the population. Estimates vary due to differences in diagnostic criteria, research methodologies, and studied populations. Here is an overview of the available data and key epidemiological factors:

1. Prevalence estimates:

➢ *Variability of estimates:*

Studies on the prevalence of MCS report varied rates, ranging from 2% to 15% of the general population. This variability is due to differences in diagnostic criteria, data collection methods, and the populations studied.

- *National and international studies:*

In the United States, studies have estimated that the prevalence of MCS is around 12% of the adult population.

In Canada, studies estimate that about 2.5% to 5% of the population reports having MCS, with a higher percentage reporting sensitivities to everyday chemicals. In 2024, this represents approximately 1 million to 2 million people affected by MCS.

In Germany, a study found that 9% of adults considered themselves sensitive to chemicals.

In Japan, a national survey estimated the prevalence at about 2% of the population.

In France, although there is no prevalence study according to ANSES (the French Agency for Food, Environmental and Occupational Health & Safety) (source: Anses; RNV3P Study Report, November 2023), a lower average estimate between Sweden and England is about 3% of the population. This figure can be applied to Spain, Portugal, Italy, and Belgium.

- *Geographic differences:*

Variations in the prevalence of MCS (Multiple Chemical Sensitivity) are also influenced by environmental, cultural, and socio-economic factors, which explains the differences observed between countries.

2. Demographic characteristics:

The prevalence of chemical sensitivity syndrome shows significant disparities based on several factors. First, it is more common in women, who account for approximately 60% to 80% of reported cases. Second, MCS tends to primarily affect middle-aged adults, with symptoms often appearing between the ages of 30 and 50. Third, individuals of lower socioeconomic status are more likely to be exposed to environmental chemicals, thereby increasing their risk of developing the condition.

3. Associated Risk Factors:

Risk factors associated with the development of MCS include primarily occupational exposure to chemicals. This includes professions such as painters, hairdressers, agricultural workers, and factory workers, who are more exposed to potential triggers. Additionally, lifestyle habits such as frequent use of household chemicals like cleaners and perfumes, as well as living in highly polluted environments, also increase the risk of developing this condition. Finally, medical history, including pre-existing allergies, asthma, and autoimmune disorders, makes individuals more susceptible to chemical sensitivities.

4. Socio-Economic Impact:

Chemical sensitivity places significant burdens on the healthcare system, with high costs associated with medical consultations, diagnostic tests, and treatments needed to manage symptoms. At the same time, it has a devastating impact on the quality of life for affected individuals, limiting their daily activities, reducing their productivity at work, and exacerbating issues of anxiety and depression. Furthermore, MCS leads to high rates of absenteeism and work disability, resulting in substantial economic repercussions for both the affected individuals and society as a whole.

5. Limitations of epidemiological data:

MCS presents several research challenges. First, the variability in diagnostic criteria complicates the comparison of studies and the establishment of accurate prevalence rates, given the lack of universally accepted criteria. Second, data on chemical sensitivity are often biased by voluntary reporting, where individuals with sensitivities are more likely to participate in surveys, potentially inflating prevalence estimates. Additionally, there is a critical lack of longitudinal data tracking individuals over long periods, which limits the understanding of the progression of MCS and its long-term impact on health.

The prevalence of chemical sensitivity varies across studies and populations, affecting a significant proportion of the population, particularly women and middle-aged adults. Risk factors include occupational exposure, lifestyle habits, and medical history. MCS has a very significant socio-economic impact, affecting quality of life and leading to high costs for the healthcare system. Further research is needed to standardize diagnostic criteria and obtain accurate epidemiological data.

1.7 Impact on quality of life

MCS has a profound and varied impact on the quality of life for those affected. The effects of this condition extend beyond physical symptoms, also affecting emotional, social, and professional aspects of life. Here is a detailed exploration of the impact of the condition on quality of life:

1. Physical impact:

Individuals with MCS endure disabling symptoms including headaches, chronic fatigue, muscle and joint pain, respiratory problems, and gastrointestinal issues, which limit their ability to perform normal daily activities. To avoid triggers, these individuals often have to restrict their exposure to certain environments, such as shopping centers, offices, and public transportation, where chemicals are present. Additionally, MCS is frequently associated with other medical conditions such as asthma, allergies, and autoimmune disorders, further complicating the management of their health.

2. Emotional and psychological impact:

The uncertainty and unpredictability of chemical triggers often lead to constant stress and anxiety for those affected. They develop an intense fear of environments that may contain chemicals. Additionally, social isolation and the limitations imposed by MCS contribute to feelings of depression. The loss of control over their environment and the reduction in enjoyable activities exacerbate this depressive state. Finally, individuals face stigma and skepticism from others, including healthcare professionals, colleagues, and even family members, which profoundly affects their emotional well-being.

3. Social impact:

Avoiding environments potentially contaminated by chemicals leads to social isolation for individuals with MCS. They limit their social interactions, which reduces their social support and increases feelings of loneliness. MCS also affects personal relationships, as close ones may not understand the severity of the condition or the need for the precautions taken by the sensitive individual, leading to tensions and conflicts. Additionally, individuals often have to give up recreational activities they previously enjoyed, such as attending social events, participating in sports, or traveling, due to the presence of chemical triggers.

4. Professional mpact:

Modern work environments, often filled with toxic substances such as cleaning products, perfumes, and building materials, can be intolerable for individuals with MCS. This limits their career options and often makes it difficult to maintain stable employment. The symptoms lead to frequent absenteeism and reduced productivity at work, forcing individuals to take extended medical leave or work part-time. Some people are compelled to change careers or seek jobs in controlled environments free of chemicals, often at significant personal and financial sacrifices.

5. Economic impact:

Managing MCS involves high medical costs, including consultations, diagnostic tests, treatments, and medications. Additionally, modifying the home environment to minimize exposure to chemicals is expensive. Professional limitations and the inability to work lead to significant loss of income, affecting the financial stability of affected individuals and their families. Furthermore, individuals incur extra expenses for specialized chemical-free products, air filters, and other necessary equipment to create a safe environment.

Many individuals are unable to continue working and are forced to stay at home, seeking financial aid from the state or, in the best cases, having their condition recognized by insurance or through legal channels to receive supplementary income from company benefits. Unfortunately, these cases are rare, and most people live on minimal social benefits that are provided to them.

Chemical sensitivity has a significant impact on quality of life, affecting numerous physical, emotional, social, professional, and economic aspects. Improved recognition and understanding of MCS, along with appropriate support, are essential for enhancing the lives of those affected. Ongoing awareness and research are crucial for developing effective management and treatment approaches.

MCS

Dr. William Rea

(1935-2018)

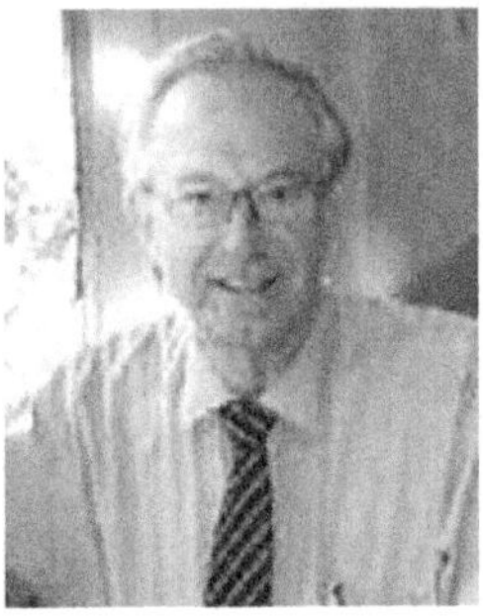

Dr. William Rea was an American physician and allergist, also known for his work in the field of environmental medicine. He was a renowned advocate for environmental treatments for patients suffering from multiple chemical sensitivities and other environment-related disorders. He founded the Environmental Health Center (EHC) in Dallas, Texas, where he developed innovative approaches to diagnose and treat illnesses caused or exacerbated by exposure to chemicals and environmental factors.

Chapter 2
A day in the life

2.1 The difficult awakening

For a person with MCS, each day often begins with a challenge. The difficult awakening is a daily reality that highlights the many obstacles these individuals face from the moment they wake up. Here is a detailed description of what a difficult awakening can represent.

1. The previous night:

People often experience difficulties obtaining restorative sleep due to various factors such as physical pain, headaches, and general discomfort caused by chemical sensitivities. Toxic products present in mattresses, sheets, or even the air in the room can disrupt sleep. Special precautions often need to be taken the night before to minimize exposure to chemicals during sleep. This includes using air purifiers, hypoallergenic bedding, and avoiding any scented or harsh cleaning products before going to bed.

2. The awakening:

Despite a night of sleep, persistent chronic fatigue is a common complaint upon waking, accompanied by a feeling of heaviness and exhaustion that makes getting out of bed difficult. Many people also wake up with joint pain, muscle stiffness, and headaches, often exacerbated by poor sleep posture or reactions to chemicals present in their sleeping environment. Upon waking, immediate symptoms such as nausea, dizziness, and brain fog may appear, often triggered by nighttime exposure to invisible yet present toxic products in the air or surrounding objects.

3. The morning routine:

Before getting out of bed, some individuals must take precautions to ensure their environment is safe. This includes ventilating the room to remove potential contaminants and using air purifiers to reduce pollutant levels. Personal care products used should be carefully selected to avoid any triggers, often favoring natural, fragrance-free, and hypoallergenic options. Regarding diet, breakfast needs to be specifically tailored, as certain foods or drinks may contain additives that trigger symptoms, necessitating a strict and controlled diet.

4. Psychological challenges:

Anxiety related to the simple act of getting up is common among those affected, exacerbated by the fear of impending symptoms or unexpected exposure to toxic products. This anticipation creates psychological tension from the start of the day. Additionally, managing energy is crucial due to the persistent fatigue and constant pain associated with MCS. Individuals must carefully plan their day, incorporating frequent breaks and rest periods to manage their energy levels effectively.

5. Coping strategies:

To minimize risks associated with chemical sensitivity, it is essential to establish a strict routine that includes specific practices for ventilating the home, preparing meals, and using personal care products. Support from family and friends plays a crucial role, allowing for the sharing or delegation of some morning tasks to ease the burden on the affected individual. Incorporating relaxation techniques such as meditation, deep breathing, and gentle yoga into the morning routine is also recommended to help manage stress and associated anxiety.

The difficult awakening is a major component of daily life for those affected, marked by persistent fatigue, pain, and vigilance to avoid chemical triggers. Coping strategies and support from those around them are essential to improving quality of life despite the constraints of MCS.

2.2 Hygiene, a challenge

Maintaining a personal hygiene routine is a significant challenge. Personal care products, detergents, and standard cleaning methods often contain toxic substances that can trigger severe symptoms. Here is a detailed exploration of the obstacles and strategies for managing daily hygiene.

1. Choosing personal care products:

To minimize reactions related to multiple chemical sensitivity, it is recommended to avoid personal care products containing synthetic fragrances, opting for those labeled "fragrance-free" or "hypoallergenic." Choosing products with natural ingredients such as Castile soap, pure organic essential oils, and organic shampoos is preferable, although even these natural ingredients can cause reactions in highly sensitive individuals. Additionally, it is advisable to avoid preservatives like parabens and artificial colorants, favoring products free from these additives.

2. Shower and bath routine:

To minimize skin reactions related to chemical sensitivity, it is recommended to use a shower filter to remove chlorine and other contaminants from the water, which can exacerbate symptoms. It is also advisable to pay attention to the water temperature, avoiding water that is too hot as it increases skin sensitivity and can cause irritation. Finally, it is best to limit the duration of showers or baths to reduce exposure to chemically treated water and steam, which contain irritants.

3. Hair care:

To care for sensitive hair, it is recommended to use shampoos and conditioners free from sulfates, silicones, and other harsh chemicals, favoring organic and natural options. Reducing the frequency of washing is advised to limit exposure to hair products, with alternatives such as "no-poo" (shampoo-free) methods or rinses using diluted apple cider vinegar.

4. Skin care:

For a safe skincare routine, it is recommended to use simple moisturizers and lotions containing natural ingredients like shea butter, coconut oil, or aloe vera. Multi-purpose products are often preferred to reduce the number of products used. It is also important to avoid common irritants such as petroleum jelly and paraffin, which clog pores and contain chemical contaminants.

5. Clothing and bedding maintenance:

To maintain a safe laundry environment, it is recommended to use mild detergents free from fragrances, dyes, and other harsh chemicals, such as soap nuts and Castile soap-based detergents. It is essential to rinse clothes and bedding several times to remove all detergent residues. Avoiding scented fabric softeners and dryer sheets, which contain irritating toxic substances, is crucial. Instead, opting for natural alternatives like wool dryer balls is recommended.

6. House cleaning:

To maintain a safe home environment, it is crucial to opt for natural cleaning products such as white vinegar, baking soda, and lemon juice, avoiding harsh chemicals found in commercial cleaners. Proper ventilation of the home is also essential to remove indoor pollutants, supported by the use of air purifiers equipped with HEPA filters. Minimizing sources of pollutants is vital by eliminating the use of scented candles, incense, and air fresheners, as these products can release toxic substances into the air that may trigger unwanted symptoms.

Personal hygiene and home maintenance present significant challenges. Carefully selecting products, adjusting routines, and creating a safe environment are essential. Despite the restrictions, strategies and alternatives allow for maintaining adequate personal hygiene while minimizing the risks of chemical reactions.

2.3 Breakfast

For a person with MCS, breakfast requires special attention to food selection and meal preparation. Food sensitivities, chemical additives, and environmental contaminants all play a role in planning this important meal of the day. Here is a detailed description of the considerations and strategies for managing breakfast.

1. Food selection:

Principles for a safe breakfast include choosing organic foods such as fruits, vegetables, grains, and dairy products to limit exposure to pesticides. Opting for whole, unprocessed foods, such as fresh fruits, pasture-raised eggs, and unsalted nuts, helps avoid additives and preservatives. It is essential to identify and avoid common allergens such as gluten, dairy products, and nuts, as well as food additives like colorants and preservatives.

2. Meal Preparation:

Using filtered water for cooking and preparing beverages is essential to remove chemical contaminants present in tap water. A high-quality water filter can reduce levels of chlorine, heavy metals, and other impurities.

Kitchen utensils made from safe materials, such as stainless steel, cast iron, and glass, are preferred. Non-stick coatings and plastics release harmful toxic substances when heated.

Gentle cooking methods such as steaming, poaching, and simmering are used to preserve the quality of foods and avoid the formation of potentially harmful chemical compounds that can appear at high temperatures.

3. Examples of suitable breakfasts:

- *Fruit smoothie:* Make a homemade smoothie with organic fruits such as bananas, berries, and apples. You can also add ground chia or flax seeds to boost the fiber and omega-3 fatty acid content.

- *Gluten-free fruit pancakes:* Make pancakes with gluten-free flour (such as almond flour or buckwheat flour), organic eggs, unsweetened plant-based milk, and a touch of vanilla. Serve with fresh fruits like banana slices, berries, or apple slices. Add pure maple syrup to sweeten to your taste.

- *Quinoa porridge with dried fruits:* Cook quinoa in unsweetened plant-based milk with dried fruits like raisins, dried apricots, or prunes. Add a pinch of cinnamon and a touch of organic honey for a slight sweetness.

- *Oat flake and fruit pancakes:* Make pancakes using oat flakes (blended into flour), organic eggs, unsweetened plant-based milk, and a touch of baking powder. Top with banana slices, fresh berries, or apple slices. Add chopped nuts and organic honey for an extra touch of flavor.

4. Managing beverages:

Recommended beverages include pure filtered water and herbal infusions like chamomile and peppermint, thus avoiding sugary drinks, commercial fruit juices, and products containing artificial additives. For tea and coffee, it is advisable to choose organic versions and monitor individual reactions. Using unbleached coffee filters and loose-leaf tea without additives is recommended to reduce exposure to potential chemicals.

5. Meal environment:

A well-ventilated kitchen is essential to eliminate potential cooking fumes. By opening windows or using a range hood, you can maintain fresh and healthy air. Additionally, it is crucial to clean food preparation surfaces with natural, non-toxic products to avoid harmful residues. Diluted white vinegar and baking soda are effective and safe choices to ensure clean and secure surfaces for meal preparation.

Breakfast requires careful planning and attention to detail. Selecting foods carefully, preparing them with care, and creating a safe meal environment are essential to avoid chemical triggers. Despite the constraints, it is possible to prepare nutritious and delicious meals that meet specific needs, thereby contributing to overall well-being.

2.4 Preparing the day

Preparing for the day involves a series of careful precautions and strategies to minimize exposure to chemicals. Here is a detailed description of the steps and considerations needed to effectively prepare for facing the day.

1. Choosing clothes:

Choosing clothing made from natural fibers like organic cotton, linen, and untreated wool is recommended to minimize chemical residues from manufacturing processes. Before wearing new clothes, it is essential to wash them several times to remove toxic finishing products such as softeners, flame retardants, and residual dyes. Avoiding garments treated with specific products like stain or antibacterial treatments is also crucial, as these treatments release irritating compounds.

2. Preparing the bag:

A "survival kit" for MCS is essential and should include FFP2 KN95 or activated charcoal respirators, cotton gloves, and unscented wipes to handle unexpected chemical exposures. Carrying safe snacks such as organic fruits, unsalted nuts, and additive-free energy bars, along with filtered water, is crucial to avoid potentially contaminated foods outside. It is also important to have prescribed medications and necessary supplements on hand to manage symptoms, such as antihistamines or anti-inflammatory drugs, in case of sudden reactions.

3. Time management:

Planning travel should include routes and modes of transport aimed at minimizing exposure to chemicals. Opting for personal car trips equipped with an activated charcoal pollen filter is often safer than public transportation. It is also essential to schedule regular breaks in controlled and safe environments to reduce cumulative exposure to toxic substances throughout the day. These breaks allow for relaxation, drinking water, and consuming safe foods. Additionally, if possible, organizing the workspace to minimize chemical exposure is recommended. This can include using an air purifier, requesting to work in an area away from printers or cleaning products, and informing colleagues about chemical sensitivity to avoid strong perfumes or sprays around oneself.

4. Stress management strategies:

Incorporating relaxation techniques into your morning routine is essential for mentally and physically preparing for the day ahead. This can include meditation, deep breathing, or light stretching. Maintaining regular contact with friends and family members who understand MCS and offer emotional support is also crucial, whether through phone calls, messages, or meetings in safe environments. Finally, having an emergency plan in case of unexpected exposure is indispensable. This involves knowing where to find immediate relief, knowing who to contact in an emergency, and having quick access to necessary medications or care products.

5. Mental and emotional preparation:

Cultivating a positive and resilient mindset is crucial for managing chemical sensitivity. This involves focusing on the controllable aspects of the day and practicing gratitude by noting small victories and pleasant moments. Simultaneously, adopting a flexible approach allows for handling unforeseen circumstances and adjusting plans based on levels of exposure to toxic products encountered. Keeping a journal to document daily experiences, identify triggers, and evaluate the effectiveness of strategies used is also essential for refining MCS management methods and better understanding personal needs.

Preparing for the day requires meticulous organization to minimize exposure to chemicals, from choosing clothes to planning travel. By combining physical, mental, and emotional preparations, individuals can approach their day with confidence and calm, despite the unique challenges posed by their condition.

2.5 Outdoors, an obstacle course

For someone with MCS, leaving the house can become a true obstacle course. The unpredictable outdoor environment, filled with various sources of toxic products, presents a constant challenge. Here is a detailed description of the obstacles faced and strategies for managing these daily challenges.

1. Preparation before leaving:

To reduce exposure to irritating substances, it is recommended to wear covering clothing, including a hat and prescription or sunglasses, to minimize direct contact with eye surfaces and atmospheric pollutants. Using respiratory masks specifically designed to filter fine particles and chemicals in the air is also essential, with preference given to those equipped with activated carbon filters for increased protection. It is wise to have an emergency kit on hand that includes antihistamines, medications for allergic reactions, unscented wipes, and bottles of filtered water to quickly address needs in case of exposure.

2. Travel:

To minimize exposure to irritating substances, it is recommended to prefer individual modes of transportation such as walking or using a personal vehicle, in order to avoid toxic products present in public transportation, such as disinfectants, perfumes, and exhaust fumes. It is also important to plan routes that bypass industrial areas, construction sites, heavily trafficked roads, and areas with high air pollution. To maintain a safe environment inside the vehicle, using portable air purifiers is advised, while avoiding air fresheners and keeping windows closed when there is high external pollution.

3. In public spaces:

To manage MCS effectively, it is recommended to frequent outdoor public spaces such as parks rather than shopping malls or enclosed buildings where the air is often saturated with chemical particles from cleaning products and ventilation systems. By maintaining adequate social distance, one can avoid exposure to perfumes, lotions, and other personal products used by people. It is also advisable to limit time spent inside buildings and, if necessary, to choose well-ventilated or less crowded areas to reduce the risk of exposure to irritating substances.

4. Social interactions:

To facilitate the management of chemical sensitivity, it is essential to clearly inform friends, colleagues, and family members of your specific needs. Request their cooperation in avoiding the use of perfumes and chemical products in your presence. For gatherings, choose safe outdoor locations or those specifically designed to minimize exposure to triggers. Always inform hosts in advance about your particular needs before visiting their home. For social activities, prefer those that take place in natural environments or public gardens, thereby limiting exposure to potentially harmful substances.

5. Shopping and purchases:

To minimize exposure to chemicals, it is recommended to favor organic stores or farmers' markets where products are less likely to be contaminated by pesticides and toxic additives. Also, use online ordering and delivery services to avoid chemicals present in physical stores, such as indoor air fresheners and cleaning products used by staff. Shopping during off-peak hours is also advised to avoid crowds and reduce increased exposure to chemicals brought by other customers.

6. Medical and professional appointments:

To manage MCS effectively, it is essential to coordinate with healthcare professionals by informing them of the condition and requesting that they use hypoallergenic and fragrance-free products during medical appointments. It is also crucial to work in a suitable work environment with good ventilation and strict policies against the use of scented products and toxic cleaners, collaborating closely with employers to create a safe workspace. When appropriate, telecommuting is a beneficial solution to avoid exposure to potentially contaminated office environments.

Navigating outdoors is complex and requires careful preparation. Whether for travel, social interactions, or shopping, every aspect of outdoor life must be managed carefully to minimize exposure to chemicals. With thoughtful planning and precautionary measures, it is possible to reduce risks and improve quality of life despite the challenges posed by MCS.

2.6 At work or school

Managing professional or academic life involves unique challenges. Work and learning environments contain various chemicals and irritating substances. Here is a detailed description of strategies and considerations for managing MCS in these contexts.

1. Communication with administration:

To facilitate the understanding of MCS, it is essential to provide detailed information to the school or employer administration, including the nature of the condition, its specific triggers, and the measures required to create a safe environment. Presenting medical documentation that includes health recommendations from doctors or specialists is crucial to justify the necessary adjustments. It is also advisable to schedule regular meetings with the administration to assess the effectiveness of the implemented strategies and make adjustments based on evolving needs.

2. Adapting the environment:

Requesting a safe workspace or classroom involves avoiding areas with chemical use, such as copy rooms, restrooms, and cafeterias, and opting for a well-ventilated space with operable windows. The use of air purifiers equipped with HEPA filters is recommended to reduce airborne pollutants, with a request for their installation in frequently used areas. It is also advisable to prioritize hypoallergenic materials and supplies, such as odor-free office products, unbleached paper, and school supplies free of irritating substances, to minimize potential triggers of multiple chemical sensitivity.

3. Fragrance-free policy:

Establishing a fragrance-free policy is essential in the workplace or school to minimize triggers for chemical sensitivity. This involves educating colleagues and peers to avoid using perfumes, scented lotions, and fragranced hair products. Additionally, it is important to request the use of non-toxic, fragrance-free cleaning products in common areas to reduce exposure to irritating substances. Offering eco-friendly and safe alternatives for regular cleaning helps create a safer and more comfortable environment for everyone.

4. Managing breaks and meals:

Identifying safe break areas where exposure to toxic substances is minimized is crucial for sensitive individuals. Avoiding break rooms shared with microwaves or refrigerators can limit exposure to food residues and potentially irritating scents. Bringing homemade meals with safe ingredients and using glass or stainless steel containers are recommended practices to avoid food contaminants and reduce exposure to plastics, thereby contributing to a safer and more accommodating work environment for those affected.

5. Remote work and distance learning:

Negotiating remote work options to reduce exposure to potentially contaminated office environments is a key strategy for individuals sensitive to chemicals. Remote work offers greater control over one's environment and allows for minimizing toxic triggers present in traditional workspaces. Additionally, considering online learning programs for students is beneficial for limiting exposure to chemicals in educational institutions. Online educational platforms provide flexible and adaptable alternatives that promote a safer and more comfortable learning environment for those affected.

6. Support from colleagues and peers:

Organizing awareness sessions to inform colleagues or classmates about multiple chemical sensitivity, its symptoms, and the steps to provide appropriate support is crucial. This awareness fosters a more understanding and cooperative environment. Additionally, creating or joining support networks within the school or workplace helps build allies who understand MCS, making it easier to navigate daily challenges and providing essential moral support.

7. Personal coping strategies:

To better manage MCS at work or school, it is essential to practice stress management techniques such as meditation, deep breathing, or yoga, which help reduce physical reactions to chemical triggers. Keeping a symptom diary is also crucial for identifying specific triggers encountered, making it easier to adapt management strategies and discuss them with administration. Additionally, establishing an emergency plan for severe reactions is recommended, which includes knowing emergency exits, informing a trusted colleague or friend about the steps to take, and having quick access to emergency medication.

Navigating work or school environments with chemical sensitivity requires thorough preparation and close collaboration with administration and colleagues. By clearly communicating needs, adapting the environment, and employing personal coping strategies, individuals create safer and more manageable conditions for their professional and academic life. Despite numerous challenges, such appropriate measures significantly enhance quality of life and productivity in these contexts.

2.7 Shopping and health consultations

Daily activities such as shopping or attending medical appointments require specific planning and vigilance to minimize exposure to chemicals. Here is a detailed description of strategies and precautions to manage these tasks effectively.

1. Grocery shopping:

To minimize exposure to chemicals while grocery shopping, it is recommended to choose organic stores or farmers' markets where products are less likely to be contaminated by pesticides and chemical additives. Opting for local stores and small grocers allows for better communication of specific needs and potentially reduces exposure to toxic products. Shopping during off-peak hours, such as early in the morning or late in the evening, helps avoid crowds and reduces exposure to perfumes and synthetic products brought by other customers. Preparing a detailed and organized shopping list by sections limits time spent in the store and avoids retracing your steps. Choosing products with secure packaging, such as glass or stainless steel, helps avoid exposure to plastics and chemical coatings. Finally, it is advisable to avoid aisles containing cleaning products, air fresheners, and perfumes that release irritating volatile substances.

2. Strategies during shopping:

To minimize exposure to chemicals during outings and shopping, it is recommended to wear a respiratory mask and cotton gloves to filter out toxic particles and reduce contact with contaminated surfaces. Additionally, wearing long-sleeved clothing and pants helps limit skin exposure to chemical residues. Using reusable shopping bags made of natural fabric, which are washed regularly, helps avoid contamination from toxic residues on plastic bags. Finally, to sanitize payment surfaces such as card terminals and basket handles, using unscented wipes to clean them before use is recommended to reduce the risk of chemical exposure.

3. Managing health appointments:

To maximize comfort and minimize risks related to MCS during medical visits, it is essential to choose healthcare professionals who are informed about MCS, including dentists, general practitioners, specialists, and therapists, and who are willing to adapt their practices to reduce chemical exposure. It is recommended to inform the medical office in advance about your chemical sensitivity to allow for preventive measures, such as using fragrance-free cleaning products and reducing perfumes in the environment. Scheduling appointments early in the morning helps avoid residues from cleaning and a higher number of patients. To limit exposure, it is preferable to wait outside or in a well-ventilated area until the healthcare professional is ready to see you, thereby minimizing exposure in the waiting room.

4. Pharmacies and health products:

Choosing pharmacies knowledgeable about Chemical Sensitivity is crucial for finding alternatives without harmful chemicals. It is advisable to discuss with the pharmacist the excipients and additives present in prescribed medications to ensure they do not contain irritating substances. Opting for natural and organic health products, such as dietary supplements, vitamins, and over-the-counter medications, is recommended to avoid artificial colors, preservatives, and flavors that can trigger reactions in individuals with MCS.

5. Alternative and online solutions:

Using online ordering and delivery services is a key strategy to avoid in-store exposures by choosing platforms that offer organic and chemical-free products. It is advisable to request that deliveries be left outside to limit direct contact with delivery personnel and to facilitate potential decontamination of packaging before bringing it into the home. Joining support groups or local cooperatives for people with sensitivities also allows for sharing resources, advice, and potentially making bulk purchases of safe products.

Grocery shopping and managing health appointments can be challenging. With careful planning, judicious choices of suppliers and healthcare professionals, and personal protection strategies, it is possible to reduce exposure to toxic products and manage these essential activities. These measures minimize the risk of reactions and promote a better quality of life.

2.8 Returning home

Returning home after a day out requires special precautions to avoid introducing contaminants into a controlled and secure environment. Here is a detailed description of the steps and strategies for effectively managing your return home.

1. Smooth transition:

Establishing a homecoming routine is essential, incorporating specific steps for decontamination and relaxation to reduce anxiety and facilitate the transition to a safe environment. This includes creating a decontamination area near the entrance of the home, equipped with a bench, a floor mat, and storage bins for clothes and shoes worn outside.

2. Decontaminating clothes and objects:

After returning home, it is recommended to immediately change out of the clothes worn outside and place them in a fabric bag or a designated laundry basket for decontamination. Then, change into clean clothes reserved specifically for home use. Next, take a quick shower to remove any chemical residues potentially present on the skin and hair, using fragrance-free and hypoallergenic toiletries. Finally, disinfect personal items such as keys, phone, and glasses with fragrance-free wipes or a damp cloth.

3. Managing groceries and brought items:

When unpacking groceries, it is advisable to do so in a well-ventilated area or outside if possible. It is also recommended to wipe down product packaging with fragrance-free wipes or a damp cloth before storing them. For cleaning the surfaces used, it is preferable to use non-toxic, fragrance-free cleaning products, such as diluted white vinegar solutions or baking soda, which provide a natural and safe option.

4. Indoor air purification:

It is essential to ensure good ventilation in the home by regularly opening windows to allow fresh air circulation. If necessary, using fans can help enhance this airflow. Additionally, operating air purifiers equipped with HEPA filters is recommended to remove residual chemical particles and maintain better indoor air quality.

5. Relaxation and recovery:

After a day spent outside, it is crucial to allocate time for relaxation and recovery. This can include engaging in calming activities such as meditation, reading, or listening to soothing music. Additionally, using relaxation techniques such as deep breathing, yoga, or stretching helps reduce stress and calm the nervous system, promoting optimal rest.

6. Logbook:

To better manage MCS, it is recommended to keep a logbook to record daily activities, locations visited, and symptoms experienced. This helps identify potential triggers and adjust management strategies accordingly. Using this information to reflect on effective strategies or those needing adjustments is essential. Collaborating with healthcare professionals to adapt treatments and preventive measures based on observations made in the logbook contributes to optimizing symptom control and relief.

7. Preparation for the next day:

To prevent the effects of multiple chemical sensitivity, it is essential to organize clothing by washing it with fragrance-free detergents and rinsing thoroughly to remove any potentially irritating residues. Additionally, carefully planning future activities by avoiding high-risk areas and scheduling regular breaks in safe environments can significantly reduce exposure to toxic products, contributing to a more comfortable and secure environment.

Returning home is crucial for reducing the risk of contamination. By using decontamination routines, non-toxic products, and relaxation techniques, one creates a healthy and calming space. Careful planning and effective strategies help manage MCS and improve daily quality of life.

2.9 Limited leisure activities

Leisure activities present significant challenges due to the pervasive presence of chemicals in many environments. However, with appropriate precautions and careful planning, it is possible to find safe and enjoyable ways to relax and entertain oneself. Here is an exploration of limited leisure activities and strategies to make them more accessible.

1. Choosing safe leisure activities:

For outdoor activities such as hiking and walking, it is advisable to choose areas away from sources of pollution and pesticides to minimize exposure to chemicals. Organic gardening, which uses natural techniques and avoids toxic products, is also recommended for individuals with MCS.

For arts and crafts, using hypoallergenic and non-toxic art materials is essential for safely engaging in activities such as painting, drawing, or other visual arts. Similarly, participating in craft activities like sewing, knitting, or DIY projects with safe, chemical-free materials is beneficial to avoid triggers.

For relaxation, reading books, magazines, or online articles is an excellent entertainment alternative with no risk of chemical exposure. Writing, whether keeping a personal journal, writing letters, or working on creative writing projects, is another enriching and safe activity for individuals with MCS.

2. Adapting social leisure activities:

Organizing social gatherings outdoors, such as picnics or meetings in parks, helps avoid exposure to chemicals found in indoor spaces, which is particularly beneficial for sensitive individuals. When inviting friends over to your home, ensure they are informed about MCS and encourage them to avoid bringing fragranced products or wearing clothes washed with scented detergents to maintain a safe and comfortable environment. To maintain social connections without exposure risks, using technologies like video conferencing and phone calls is a practical and safe alternative.

3. Cultural and recreational activities:

To recreate a cinematic or theatrical experience at home, it is advisable to watch recorded movies or plays, thereby avoiding potentially problematic cinemas and theaters. Additionally, participating in virtual tours of museums, art galleries, and historical sites allows for cultural and educational enrichment without leaving the house, providing a safe and enjoyable alternative.

4. Physical activities and well-being:

To maintain physical activity while minimizing exposure to triggers, it is recommended to engage in home exercises such as yoga, pilates, or fitness workouts using online videos or mobile apps. For those who prefer outdoor activities, participating in sports like cycling, swimming in natural pools, or tai-chi[3] in controlled environments away from pollution sources is beneficial for health while reducing risks associated with chemical sensitivity.

5. Preparation and equipment:

To minimize exposure to chemicals and enhance safety during outdoor activities, it is advisable to use protective

3 Tai-chi is an ancient Chinese practice that combines slow movements, deep breathing, and meditation. It improves balance, flexibility, muscle strength, and reduces stress, making it accessible to all ages.

equipment such as respirator masks and long clothing. For creative and artistic activities, opting for hypoallergenic and chemical-free materials is recommended. Additionally, carefully planning outings and activities by checking environmental conditions and choosing times when pollution is minimal can reduce risks.

6. Creating a home environment suitable for hobbies:

To improve the quality of life at home for affected individuals, it is recommended to set up a leisure space equipped with air purifiers and safe materials, dedicated to creative, physical, and relaxation activities. Additionally, investing in technologies such as e-book readers, home theater systems, and streaming[4] devices can diversify the entertainment options available at home.

Hobbies require adjustments, but it is possible to enjoy enriching activities. By choosing suitable activities, safe materials, and planning outings, health risks can be minimized. Creating a secure home environment and promoting outdoor activities in controlled areas maintain a balance between relaxation, socialization, and well-being.

2.10 Evening and sleep

The evening and preparation for sleep are crucial times to relax and rejuvenate the body after a day of potential exposure to various chemical triggers. A well-planned routine and specific strategies help create a safe and conducive environment for restful sleep. Here is a detailed description of the steps and precautions to take for effectively managing the evening and sleep.

4 Streaming allows you to view or listen to multimedia content in real-time over the internet without downloading it.

1. Transitioning to the evening:

To improve sleep quality, it is essential to establish an evening routine that includes relaxing activities such as reading, listening to soothing music, or meditating to signal to the body that it's time to unwind. It is also recommended to prepare a light dinner with organic and unprocessed foods, eaten at least two hours before bedtime, to promote optimal digestion and avoid food reactions that could disrupt sleep.

2. Preparing the bedroom:

To improve the sleep environment, it is recommended to ventilate the room by opening the windows during the day to refresh the air and reduce indoor pollutant levels. Using air purifiers with HEPA filters also helps maintain optimal air quality. Additionally, opting for hypoallergenic bedding and pillows made from organic cotton or natural materials avoids irritations caused by synthetic materials containing chemicals. Finally, it is important to regularly clean the room with non-toxic, fragrance-free products, favoring natural solutions such as diluted white vinegar and baking soda to maintain a clean and healthy environment.

3. Personal hygiene:

To enhance comfort and reduce symptoms, it is advisable to use fragrance-free and hypoallergenic personal care products during the evening shower, avoiding those containing parabens, sulfates, and artificial colors. Additionally, establishing a decontamination routine by taking a shower before bedtime helps remove chemical residues accumulated on the skin and hair after a day outdoors, which contributes to reducing reactions and promoting more restful sleep.

4. Relaxing activities:

To improve sleep quality, it is recommended to practice relaxation techniques such as meditation, deep breathing, or gentle yoga to calm the mind and relax the body before bedtime. Additionally, reading books or listening to audiobooks with soothing content promotes relaxation. It is crucial to avoid exposure to bright screens, as this disrupts the sleep cycle. These practices help create a sleep-friendly environment and enhance the quality of nighttime rest.

5. Managing light and noise:

To optimize the sleep environment, it is recommended to use dim lighting or adjustable lamps to create a relaxing atmosphere in the bedroom. Avoid exposure to blue light from electronic screens, which disrupts melatonin[5] production, a hormone important for sleep. Additionally, it is essential to ensure good soundproofing in the room to minimize noise disturbances. This can be achieved by using thick, non-synthetic curtains, natural rugs, or earplugs if necessary, to foster an environment conducive to better quality sleep.

6. Optimal sleep environment:

To promote better sleep quality, it is recommended to invest in a high-quality mattress made from natural and hypoallergenic materials. Additionally, regularly changing bed linens is advised to maintain a clean environment free from allergens. It is also important to maintain a comfortable ambient temperature in the bedroom, typically between 18 and 21 degrees Celsius, to encourage deep and

5 Melatonin is a hormone produced by the pineal gland that regulates the sleep-wake cycle. When used as a supplement, it helps treat sleep disorders and jet lag.

restorative sleep. These adjustments help minimize sleep disturbances and enhance the quality of rest.

7. Monitoring and follow-up:

To improve sleep quality, it is recommended to keep a sleep journal to track sleep habits, nighttime awakenings, and disruptive factors. This helps identify potential triggers and adjust the sleep routine accordingly. If issues persist, it is essential to consult a healthcare professional to explore tailored solutions for MCS, such as medical interventions or lifestyle adjustments, aimed at optimizing nighttime rest and reducing the impact of symptoms on overall quality of life.

Managing the evening and sleep requires careful preparation. By establishing a calming routine, using hypoallergenic products, and creating an optimal sleep environment, one can minimize disruptions from chemical triggers and promote restorative sleep. These measures enhance quality of life and strengthen resilience against the challenges of MCS.

MCS

Chapter 3
The impact on health

3.1 Debilitating physical symptoms

Chemical sensitivity manifests through a range of debilitating physical symptoms that significantly impact the quality of life for those affected. These symptoms vary and affect different systems of the body, often making the diagnosis and management of MCS particularly complex. Here is a detailed description of the primary physical phenomena and their impact on health.

1. Respiratory symptoms:

Exposure to chemicals can lead to various respiratory symptoms. Dyspnea, or difficulty breathing, is common even at low concentrations of chemicals and is often accompanied by a sensation of chest tightness. Chronic coughing may also occur, triggered by volatile substances such as perfumes, cleaning products, or exhaust fumes. Additionally, exposure to toxic irritants can cause inflammation of the respiratory tract, leading to sore throat, itching, and a burning sensation. These symptoms exacerbate respiratory distress and contribute to the complexity of daily management of MCS.

2. Neurological symptoms:

Exposure to chemicals can trigger a range of debilitating neurological symptoms. Headaches, including migraines, are common and are often triggered by strong odors, air pollutants, or chemicals in indoor environments. Dizziness and lightheadedness are also frequently reported, compromising balance and coordination and increasing the risk of falls and accidents. Additionally, concentration problems and cognitive disturbances, commonly referred to as "brain fog," are prevalent, significantly affecting the ability to perform daily tasks, work, or study effectively. These complex and interrelated symptoms contribute to daily distress and a reduced quality of life for individuals.

3. Skin symptoms:

Exposure to chemicals can trigger various disruptive skin symptoms. Rashes, redness, and itching are common, ranging from mild irritations to severe eruptions. In particular, contact dermatitis, an inflammatory reaction caused by direct contact with allergens or chemical irritants, leads to redness, blisters, and peeling of the skin. Additionally, some individuals may experience burning or tingling sensations on the skin when exposed to toxic products or irritating substances, contributing to overall discomfort and a deterioration in quality of life.

4. Gastrointestinal symptoms:

Individuals may experience a variety of disruptive gastrointestinal symptoms. Nausea and vomiting are common reactions to exposure to strong odors or chemicals that are inhaled or ingested. Abdominal pain and cramping also occur, often in response to toxic foods or synthetic substances in the food environment. Additionally, gastrointestinal disturbances such as diarrhea and constipation can be persistent symptoms, exacerbated by exposure to chemicals in food or drinking water, further worsening the quality of life for those affected by this complex condition.

5. Cardiovascular symptoms:

Individuals may experience several debilitating cardiovascular symptoms. Palpitations, or rapid and irregular heartbeats, are common with chemical exposure and often lead to anxiety. Additionally, some people may develop hypertension in response to chemical stress, increasing the risk of long-term cardiovascular issues. Chest pain is also reported, frequently linked to heightened anxiety due to toxic exposure, contributing to the overall distress of those affected by this complex condition.

6. Musculoskeletal symptoms:

Individuals often experience muscle and joint pain, which is exacerbated by exposure to toxic substances, making movement and physical activities difficult. Chronic fatigue is a major and debilitating symptom, limiting the ability to perform daily tasks and requiring extended periods of rest for recovery. Additionally, generalized muscle weakness may occur, making physical activities exhausting and reducing overall endurance.

Debilitating symptoms affect nearly all systems of the body, making disease management complex. Their severity and nature vary among individuals, interfering with daily activities, work, and social life. A thorough understanding of these manifestations and a proactive approach to avoiding chemical triggers are essential for improving quality of life. Personalized management strategies, developed with informed healthcare professionals, can help mitigate these symptoms and provide crucial support.

3.2 Cognitive and neurological disorders

MCS affects not only physical health but also cognitive and neurological functions. These disorders are debilitating and have a profound impact on daily life, work capacity, and social interactions. Here is a detailed description of the cognitive and neurological disorders associated with chemical sensitivity and their impact on health.

1. Memory and concentration problems:

Individuals experience memory problems, struggling to remember recent information or recall past events, which affects their ability to perform daily tasks, follow instructions, and remember important events. They also encounter concentration difficulties, making it hard to complete tasks that require sustained attention as they feel easily distracted or unable to focus on a single task for extended periods. Additionally, "brain fog" describes a sensation of mental confusion, disorientation, and fuzzy thinking, leading to challenges in thinking clearly, making decisions, and solving problems.

2. Mood disorders and anxiety:

MCS is often associated with depressive symptoms, such as a depressed mood, loss of interest in usual activities, increased fatigue, and feelings of hopelessness, exacerbated by the chronic nature of chemical sensitivity and its imposed limitations. Affected individuals frequently experience heightened anxiety, especially when anticipating potential exposure to chemicals, leading to hypervigilance and a constant fear of encountering triggers. Additionally, exposure to toxic substances can cause irritability and rapid mood swings, making individuals easily agitated or frustrated.

3. Dizziness and balance disorders:

Dizziness, or sensations of spinning, can occur with exposure to chemicals, making walking, driving, and other activities requiring good balance challenging. Balance disorders increase the risk of falls and accidents, limiting individuals' ability to move safely.

4. Headaches and migraines:

Frequent headaches, ranging from mild to severe, are common in individuals with MCS and can be triggered by exposure to various toxic substances or environmental irritants. Migraines, which can be particularly debilitating, are often associated with symptoms such as nausea, vomiting, sensitivity to light (photophobia), and sensitivity to sound (phonophobia), and can last from several hours to several days.

5. Increased sensory sensitivities:

- *Hyperesthesia:* Hyperesthesia is an increased sensitivity to sensory stimuli, including touch, sound, light, and odors. Individuals may find normally tolerable stimuli to be extremely unpleasant or painful.

- *Photophobia:* Increased sensitivity to light often causes headaches, eye discomfort, and aversion to bright environments.

- *Phonophobia:* Increased sensitivity to sound can cause discomfort or pain in response to loud or prolonged noises.

6. Impact on executive functions:

Executive functions such as planning, organization, and time management are affected by MCS, making it challenging to handle complex tasks or complete long-term projects. Additionally, cognitive impairments hinder the ability to make effective decisions, leading to difficulties in evaluating options, weighing pros and cons, and choosing the best course of action.

Cognitive and neurological disorders can be as debilitating as physical symptoms. They impact memory, concentration, mood, and executive functions, complicating daily and professional management. A multidisciplinary approach involving healthcare professionals, therapists, and counselors helps mitigate these symptoms and develop effective strategies. Understanding and recognizing these disorders is crucial for improving quality of life and providing adequate support.

3.3 Immune system exhaustion

Chemical sensitivity is not limited to physical and neurological symptoms; it can also lead to significant immune system exhaustion. This weakening makes individuals more vulnerable to infections and other illnesses, worsening their overall health condition. In this section, we will explore the aspects of immune system exhaustion associated with MCS, its manifestations, and possible strategies for managing it.

1. Functioning of the immune system:

The immune system is responsible for protecting the body against infections, diseases, and foreign substances, comprising a variety of cells and mechanisms that identify and neutralize pathogens. In a healthy immune system, immune cells respond to invaders such as bacteria, viruses, and toxins by attacking and eliminating them effectively, with a regulated and proportional response to the threat.

2. Impact of MCS on the immune system:

In individuals with MCS, the immune system becomes hyperreactive, overreacting to normally harmless substances, which depletes immune resources and causes chronic inflammation. Constant or repeated exposure to chemicals leads to systemic inflammation, damaging body tissues and weakening the immune response, making the body more susceptible to infections and illnesses. Additionally, MCS disrupts the normal balance of the immune system, resulting in dysfunction that may manifest as reduced ability to fight infections or an increased tendency to develop autoimmune diseases.

3. Manifestations of immune system exhaustion:

- *Frequent infections:* Individuals experience frequent infections, such as colds, respiratory infections, skin infections, and other infectious diseases. This is due to a weakened immune system that is unable to respond effectively.

- *Slow recovery:* Recovery from an infection or illness is slower in affected individuals. The body, already weakened from the constant struggle against chemicals, struggles to recover quickly.

- *Chronic fatigue:* Intense chronic fatigue is often reported by individuals. This is a direct consequence of immune system exhaustion, as the body expends a significant amount of energy fighting environmental triggers.

- *Muscle and joint pain:* Muscle and joint pain is exacerbated by systemic inflammation and immune system exhaustion. This chronic pain contributes to a decline in quality of life and limits daily activities.

4. Strategies for managing immune system exhaustion:

- *Avoidance of triggers:* Minimizing exposure to chemicals and other environmental triggers is crucial. This includes measures such as using non-toxic household products, purifying indoor air, and consuming organic foods.

- *Strengthening the immune system:* Adopting a healthy lifestyle to boost the immune system. This includes a balanced diet rich in antioxidants, vitamins, and minerals, as well as integrating immune-boosting supplements if necessary.

- *Stress management:* Chronic stress further weakens the immune system. Stress management techniques, such as meditation, yoga, and deep breathing, help reduce the impact of stress on the body.

- *Physical exercise:* Regular, moderate physical activity strengthens the immune system and improves resistance to infections. However, it is important to avoid overexertion, which could worsen fatigue.

- *Restorative sleep:* Quality sleep is essential for recovery and immune system reinforcement. Establishing a regular sleep routine and creating a sleep-friendly environment enhance the quality of rest.

- *Medical consultation:* Work closely with healthcare professionals to monitor immune function and manage symptoms. Doctors can recommend specific tests and tailored treatments to support the immune system.

Immune System Exhaustion is a major aspect of chemical sensitivity, contributing to increased susceptibility to infections and prolonged recovery times. Effective management of this exhaustion requires a holistic approach that includes avoiding chemical triggers, strengthening the immune system, managing stress, and receiving appropriate medical care. By adopting these strategies, individuals can improve their quality of life and reduce the negative impacts of MCS on their immune health.

3.4 Frequent comorbidities

MCS is often associated with various comorbidities, which are medical conditions that coexist with chemical sensitivity and exacerbate the symptoms or make their management more complex. Understanding these comorbidities is essential for providing comprehensive and effective care to affected individuals. Here is a detailed exploration of common comorbidities associated with MCS.

1. Chronic fatigue syndrome (CFS):

Chronic Fatigue Syndrome is a condition characterized by severe and persistent fatigue that is not relieved by rest and interferes with daily activities. Symptoms include muscle pain, sleep disturbances, memory and concentration problems, and headaches. Chronic fatigue is a common symptom in people with Multiple Chemical Sensitivity, and the two conditions can overlap. Chronic inflammation and immune exhaustion associated with MCS contribute to the development or worsening of Chronic Fatigue Syndrome.

2. Fibromyalgia:

Fibromyalgia is a condition characterized by widespread muscle pain, increased sensitivity to pressure points, and chronic fatigue. Affected individuals may also experience sleep disturbances, headaches, and problems with memory and concentration. Fibromyalgia and MCS share many common symptoms, such as pain and fatigue. Nervous system hyperreactivity and chronic inflammation play a role in both conditions, and it is not uncommon for individuals with chemical sensitivity to also be diagnosed with fibromyalgia.

3. Irritable Bowel Syndrome (IBS):

Irritable Bowel Syndrome (IBS) is a functional gastrointestinal disorder characterized by abdominal pain, bloating, and changes in bowel habits, such as diarrhea or constipation. Individuals with Chemical Sensitivity are more sensitive to foods and chemical additives, which can exacerbate IBS symptoms. Additionally, systemic inflammation and immune dysfunction associated with MCS are likely to contribute to intestinal sensitivity.

4. Anxiety and depressive disorders:

Anxiety disorders, such as generalized anxiety, phobias, and panic disorder, are characterized by excessive worry, agitation, and panic attacks, while depression is marked by a persistently low mood, loss of interest in usual activities, and feelings of hopelessness. The chronic and debilitating nature of Multiple Chemical Sensitivity significantly increases the risk of developing anxiety and depressive states in affected individuals. The uncertainty related to chemical triggers and the social isolation associated with MCS also contribute to the onset and exacerbation of these psychological issues.

5. Food allergies and intolerances:

Food allergies involve an immune system reaction to certain foods, causing symptoms such as rashes, itching, swelling, and gastrointestinal disturbances. In contrast, food intolerances lead to non-immune reactions like abdominal pain, bloating, and diarrhea. Individuals with MCS, due to their hyperreactive immune system, are more likely to develop food allergies and intolerances. Managing these symptoms often requires strict avoidance of certain foods and chemical additives to prevent adverse reactions.

6. Asthma and other respiratory diseases:

Asthma is a chronic respiratory condition characterized by inflammation of the airways, episodes of wheezing, coughing, and shortness of breath. Other respiratory diseases, such as chronic bronchitis and allergic rhinitis, share similar symptoms. Chemical irritants and environmental pollutants that trigger MCS can also exacerbate symptoms of asthma and other respiratory conditions. Due to their increased sensitivity, individuals with MCS are more vulnerable to respiratory exacerbations, requiring careful management of environmental triggers to mitigate these effects.

7. Autoimmune disorders:

Autoimmune disorders occur when the immune system attacks the body's own tissues, as seen in conditions such as lupus, rheumatoid arthritis, and Hashimoto's thyroiditis. Symptoms, including joint pain, skin rashes, and chronic fatigue, vary depending on the specific disease. Chronic inflammation and immune dysfunction associated with MCS increase the risk of developing autoimmune diseases. Therefore, close monitoring and management of environmental triggers are essential to mitigate autoimmune symptoms in individuals with MCS.

Common comorbid conditions associated with Chemical Sensitivity add complexity to its management. Understanding these related conditions and their interaction with MCS is crucial for providing integrated care and improving patient quality of life. A multidisciplinary approach involving specialists from various health fields can promote a holistic and effective management of these conditions. By identifying and addressing comorbidities, it is possible to reduce the overall disease burden and improve patient outcomes.

3.5 A vicious circle

Chemical sensitivity often generates a vicious circle of symptoms and comorbidities that feed into each other, worsening the overall condition of the affected individual. This chapter examines the dynamics of this vicious circle, how it develops and perpetuates itself, and strategies to break this destructive cycle.

1. Development of the vicious circle:

During the initial sensitization to chemicals, whether through a single high-dose exposure or repeated exposures to lower doses, a sensitization reaction is triggered, characterized by an exaggerated immune response and heightened nervous system reactivity. This increasing hyperreactivity means that the body becomes increasingly sensitive to progressively lower levels of chemicals, thereby broadening the range of potential triggers. Consequently, continued exposure to these toxic triggers, even at low levels, leads to chronic symptoms such as headaches, fatigue, muscle pain, cognitive disturbances, and persistent gastrointestinal symptoms. These constant symptoms not only weaken the body but also the mind, significantly impacting the quality of life for individuals with chemical sensitivity.

2. Exacerbation by comorbidities:

The interference of comorbidities such as chronic fatigue syndrome, fibromyalgia, and anxiety disorders complicates the management of Multiple Chemical Sensitivity, adding an additional layer of complexity and suffering. For instance, chronic fatigue exacerbates pain and chemical sensitivity, while anxiety heightens physiological reactions to chemical exposures. The symptoms of these comorbidities and those of MCS mutually reinforce each other, creating a vicious circle. For example, systemic inflammation associated with chemical sensitivity worsens the symptoms of fibromyalgia, while chronic pain increases anxiety and stress, further exacerbating chemical sensitivity symptoms. This complex interaction between different conditions makes the overall management of health for individuals with chemical sensitivity particularly challenging and requires an integrative and targeted therapeutic approach.

3. Psychological and social impact:

The social isolation of individuals with chemical sensitivity, driven by the need to avoid toxic triggers present in public environments, leads to significant psychological distress. This social withdrawal intensifies feelings of depression and anxiety, reinforcing a vicious circle. The constant stress associated with managing the condition, combined with the fear of physical reactions to toxic substances, results in chronic anxiety that, in turn, exacerbates both physical and mental symptoms. This cycle of stress and reaction contributes to the deterioration of quality of life for those with MCS, amplifying the challenges related to daily management of their condition.

4. Immune system exhaustion:

Chronic inflammation resulting from continuous exposure to chemical triggers contributes to the weakening of the immune system, making it less effective in fighting infections and increasing the risk of developing autoimmune diseases. This immune dysfunction not only exacerbates the symptoms of Chemical Sensitivity but also worsens associated comorbidities, creating a vicious circle. Additionally, a weakened immune system increases susceptibility to frequent infections, which can, in turn, trigger or worsen MCS symptoms. Each infectious episode further weakens the immune system, thereby exacerbating the disease cycle.

5. Strategies to break the vicious circle:

To manage chemical sensitivity, several approaches are essential. First, minimizing exposure to chemicals by using non-toxic household products, purifying indoor air, and choosing organic foods is crucial. Concurrently, behavioral therapies such as cognitive-behavioral therapy (CBT) help manage anxiety and stress associated with MCS, while meditation, yoga, and other relaxation techniques also contribute to overall well-being. Maintaining social connections and participating in support groups are vital for alleviating social isolation and sharing coping strategies with others affected.

Additionally, an integrative treatment plan that includes medications, supplements, physical therapies, and nutritional interventions, developed in collaboration with healthcare professionals, is crucial for managing symptoms and strengthening the immune system. Finally, educating and raising awareness among family members, employers, and healthcare professionals about MCS is necessary to create a more understanding and accommodating environment, thereby reducing stress and accidental exposures to chemical triggers.

Chemical sensitivity creates a vicious circle of hyperreactivity, chronic symptoms, and comorbidities that reinforce each other, worsening the health condition of affected individuals. To break this cycle, a holistic and multidisciplinary approach is necessary, encompassing trigger management, psychological support, immune system strengthening, and quality of life improvement. By understanding these dynamics and adopting appropriate strategies, it is possible to reduce the impact of MCS and improve overall health.

3.6 Psychological consequences

MCS has a significant impact not only on physical health but also on the mental and emotional well-being of those who suffer from it. The psychological consequences of chemical sensitivity are as debilitating as the physical symptoms, exacerbating overall suffering and complicating disease management. This section explores the various dimensions of the psychological consequences associated with MCS.

1. Chronic anxiety and stress:

Individuals with chemical sensitivity live in constant fear of chemical triggers present in their environment, which generates chronic anxiety and keeps them in a state of hypervigilance. This fear of invisible and omnipresent triggers increases daily stress and contributes to the worsening of physical symptoms associated with MCS. The chronic stress resulting from managing this condition creates a vicious circle where physical symptoms are exacerbated, further weakening the immune system and negatively affecting sleep, appetite, and mood.

2. Depression:

MCS generates a profound sense of despair in affected individuals due to its chronic and often unpredictable nature. This condition leads to feelings of helplessness and loss of control over life and health, thereby increasing the risk of developing clinical depression. Additionally, the necessary avoidance of social situations to reduce exposure to toxic substances results in significant social isolation. This social withdrawal limits interactions with others and decreases available social support, thereby reinforcing feelings of loneliness and sadness among individuals with MCS

3. Mood disorders:

Individuals with chemical sensitivity often face increased irritability and outbursts of anger due to the constant challenges of managing their condition. The frustration of not being understood or supported by others intensifies these negative emotions, which are further exacerbated by fluctuations in physical symptoms. Frequent mood changes are a direct consequence of these physiological variations: good days bring hope and temporary relief, while bad days plunge individuals into deep distress and significant frustration, further complicating the emotional management of MCS.

4. Post-traumatic stress disorder (PTSD):

For some individuals with chemical sensitivity, the initial exposure to toxic chemicals can trigger symptoms of Post-Traumatic Stress Disorder. Intrusive memories, nightmares, and stress reactions are common manifestations of this disorder, exacerbating existing symptoms related to MCS. PTSD also reinforces avoidance behaviors and hypervigilance in individuals, amplifying the fear of new exposures to chemical triggers and contributing to a cycle of increased stress and heightened reactions.

5. Emotional exhaustion:

Constant management of physical symptoms and chemical triggers associated with Multiple Chemical Sensitivity leads to intense psychological exhaustion in patients. This emotional exhaustion results in a significant decrease in energy, motivation, and ability to cope with daily challenges. As a result, individuals' coping resources are limited, affecting their ability to effectively use coping strategies. This increases their dependence on others' support and heightens their vulnerability to emotional crises.

6. Strategies for managing psychological consequences:

Managing chemical sensitivity involves a holistic approach aimed at improving both mental health and overall well-being. Cognitive-behavioral therapy (CBT) is used to address anxiety, depression, and mood disorders by focusing on modifying negative thoughts and behaviors. Relaxation techniques, such as meditation, yoga, and deep breathing, are also recommended to reduce stress and improve emotional well-being, while mindfulness helps individuals stay focused on the present moment and decrease anticipatory anxiety. Support groups play a crucial role by providing a safe space to share experiences, advice, and emotional support, thus reducing social isolation and offering practical coping strategies. Educating family members, employers, and healthcare professionals about MCS is essential for creating a supportive and understanding environment, which helps reduce stigma and improve social interactions. Finally, engaging in enjoyable activities and hobbies adapted to the environment helps improve mood and provides positive distraction, thereby fostering better emotional balance in the daily management of chemical sensitivity.

The psychological consequences of chemical sensitivity are complex and profound, affecting all aspects of the lives of those affected. Effective management of these impacts requires an integrated approach combining psychological interventions, relaxation techniques, and social support. By addressing these psychological dimensions of MCS, quality of life is improved, and better mental and emotional health is fostered.

3.7 Financial costs

Chemical sensitivity not only leads to physical and psychological consequences but also incurs significant financial costs. These expenses can quickly accumulate and become a burden for individuals and their families. This section examines the various sources of financial costs associated with MCS and offers strategies for managing them.

1. Medical care and treatments:

Individuals with chemical sensitivity face significant health-related expenses. Firstly, regular consultations with various specialists such as allergists, immunologists, neurologists, and psychiatrists are necessary for disease monitoring and symptom management, leading to substantial medical costs. Additionally, diagnostic tests to identify chemical sensitivities and comorbidities are expensive, including laboratory tests, blood analyses, allergy tests, and specialized evaluations. Moreover, the medications required to manage MCS symptoms and supplements aimed at strengthening the immune system represent ongoing expenses, varying depending on symptom severity and medical recommendations. Finally, many affected individuals turn to alternative therapies like acupuncture, homeopathy, and naturopathy, which, although potentially beneficial, are often not covered by health insurance, further increasing the overall financial burden for those with MCS.

2. Environmental adaptations:

- *Home improvements:* Environmental adaptations to minimize exposure to chemicals include installing air purifiers, using non-toxic building materials, and renovating to remove mold and other pollutants. These modifications can be costly but are often necessary to create a safe environment.

- *Specialized household products:* Purchasing non-toxic household products, including cleaning agents, cosmetics, and personal care items, increases daily expenses. These products are generally more expensive than their conventional counterparts.

- *Hypoallergenic clothing and bedding:* Individuals with chemical sensitivity require clothing and bedding made from hypoallergenic materials, which represents an additional cost.

3. Loss of income:

Individuals with chemical sensitivity face significant employment challenges. First, the symptoms of MCS often make it difficult, if not impossible, to maintain full-time employment, forcing individuals to reduce their working hours or leave their jobs entirely, resulting in a substantial loss of income. Second, some people must consider career changes to find work environments with less chemical exposure, which can lead to a decrease in salary and additional costs related to retraining and career transition. Third, frequent absences due to severe symptoms or medical appointments contribute to reduced wages, loss of bonuses, and increased job insecurity, thus affecting the financial and professional stability of individuals with MCS.

4. Family support and home care:

Daily management of MCS imposes significant financial burdens on affected individuals. First, hiring home care assistance for household tasks or personal care often becomes necessary when symptoms limit a person's autonomy, adding an additional financial cost. Second, family members may be compelled to provide financial support to cover medical expenses and necessary environmental adaptations, putting financial pressure on the entire household. Third, individuals with MCS frequently require specialized transportation services to avoid exposure to chemicals present in public transit, with these services being more costly than conventional transportation options. These financial challenges exacerbate the difficulties associated with managing MCS and highlight the urgent need for accessible financial support for patients and their families.

5. Insurance and financial assistance

The financial challenges associated with chemical sensitivity are numerous and varied. First, health insurance does not cover all aspects of the care needed for MCS, including alternative therapies and home modifications, leaving a significant portion of the costs to be borne by the patients. Second, although there are government aids and grants for people with chronic conditions, accessing these aids is often complex and requires detailed medical documentation. Third, an increasing number of patients are turning to crowdfunding[6] and community support through online platforms to obtain financial help from the community, although this option is not a long-term solution. These realities highlight the importance of increased awareness and more accessible solutions to financially support individuals with MCS in their care and management journey.

The financial costs associated with chemical sensitivity are high and represent an additional burden for affected individuals and their families. To manage them effectively, it is crucial to carefully plan finances, use available resources wisely, and seek

6 Crowdfunding is a type of participatory funding where individuals financially support a project through an online platform, allowing for the mobilization of funds without going through traditional channels.

social and community support. By identifying various sources of expenses and exploring solutions to minimize them, it is possible to reduce the financial impact of MCS and improve the quality of life for those affected.

3.8 The challenges of diagnosis

Diagnosing multiple chemical sensitivity presents numerous challenges due to the complexity and variability of its symptoms, as well as the lack of consensus within the medical community on diagnostic criteria. This section explores the main obstacles to diagnosing MCS and suggests ways to improve recognition and management of this condition.

1. Variability of symptoms:

The challenges associated with chemical sensitivity are numerous and complex. First, non-specific symptoms such as headaches, fatigue, muscle pain, digestive issues, and cognitive difficulties are often attributed to other medical conditions, making the diagnosis of MCS difficult and frequently delayed. Second, symptoms fluctuate in intensity and frequency, with periods of remission followed by sudden exacerbations, complicating the identification of clear patterns. Third, chemical sensitivity is multisystemic, affecting multiple body systems including the nervous, immune, and digestive systems, requiring a holistic and interdisciplinary approach that is often lacking in conventional healthcare. These complex characteristics of MCS highlight the need for better recognition and an integrated approach in the diagnosis and management of this controversial medical condition.

2. Lack of standardized diagnostic criteria:

To date, chemical sensitivity presents several significant diagnostic challenges. Firstly, the absence of specific and validated biomarkers makes diagnosis primarily based on clinical history and the exclusion of other medical conditions, which can lead to errors and frustration for patients. Additionally, the variability in evaluation criteria for MCS among healthcare professionals and across countries contributes to inconsistencies in assessments and a lack of official recognition of the condition. Some doctors adopt strict criteria, while others prefer a more inclusive approach, exacerbating the differences in interpretation and management. Furthermore, chemical sensitivity remains a controversial topic within the medical community, with some professionals recognizing it as a valid medical condition, while others consider it a psychosomatic or functional disorder. This divergence of opinions directly influences the evaluation and treatment processes for patients, highlighting the need for better standardization of diagnostic criteria and greater awareness in medical practice.

3. Complexity of medical history:

Identifying specific chemical exposures in patients with chemical sensitivity is complex due to the diversity of substances they encounter in their daily environment. The cumulative effects of low-dose exposures over long periods are poorly understood and challenging to assess accurately. Additionally, patients often have a complex medical history, characterized by multiple medical consultations and unsuccessful treatment attempts, making it particularly difficult for doctors to achieve a clear and unified diagnosis. Effectively integrating this heterogeneous information requires an individualized diagnostic and therapeutic approach. Moreover, psychosocial factors such as stress, anxiety, and traumatic life events play a crucial role in the onset and progression of MCS symptoms but are often under-evaluated in traditional medical consultations. A comprehensive and thorough assessment of these factors is essential for a holistic and effective management of patients with MCS.

4. Organizational and systemic obstacles:

Limited access to specialized care for chemical sensitivity presents a major challenge for many patients, who often face extended wait times to see knowledgeable healthcare professionals, sometimes located far from their homes. This situation significantly delays appropriate diagnosis and treatment, exacerbating difficulties in managing symptoms. Additionally, the high costs of diagnostic tests needed to rule out other medical conditions and confirm Multiple Chemical Sensitivity, combined with the lack of insurance coverage for many specific treatments, deter some patients from seeking comprehensive evaluation. Furthermore, the lack of specific training on MCS in healthcare professionals' educational programs contributes to a lack of awareness of this condition, leading to its prevalence being underestimated and inadequate management by practitioners. To improve the situation, it is crucial to enhance access to specialized care, reduce financial barriers to tests and treatments, and integrate more information about MCS into ongoing medical education to improve recognition and management of this complex condition.

5. Strategies to improve diagnosis:

To improve the recognition and management of Multiple Chemical Sensitivity, several measures are essential. It is crucial to develop standardized and internationally recognized diagnostic criteria to standardize the diagnostic process. Simultaneously, research on potential biomarkers should be encouraged to develop more objective and reliable diagnostic tests. Enhancing the understanding of MCS among healthcare professionals requires the integration of specific modules into medical training programs and the organization of awareness workshops. A multidisciplinary approach involving allergists, immunologists, neurologists, psychiatrists, and psychologists is also recommended for a comprehensive patient evaluation. Finally, improving access to specialized care and diagnostic tests through government grants or financial assistance programs would help patients obtain an early diagnosis and appropriate treatment.

The challenges of diagnosing Multiple Chemical Sensitivity are numerous and complex, ranging from symptom variability to the lack of standardized diagnostic criteria. To advance, it is crucial to develop uniform diagnostic criteria, research biomarkers, enhance healthcare professional training, and promote a multidisciplinary approach. By adopting these strategies, we can improve the recognition, diagnosis, and management of MCS, thereby reducing patient suffering and improving their quality of life.

MCS

Chapter 4
Diagnosing chemical sensitivity

4.1 Absence of specific tests

Diagnosing chemical sensitivity represents a major challenge due to the absence of validated specific tests. This section examines the implications of this absence and explores the current approaches used to diagnose MCS.

1. Problems related to the absence of specific tests:

The diagnosis of multiple chemical sensitivity primarily relies on the exclusion of other medical conditions with similar symptoms, such as allergies, food intolerances, autoimmune diseases, and psychiatric disorders, due to the absence of dedicated specific tests. This exclusion process is often lengthy and frustrating for patients, thus delaying the implementation of appropriate treatment. The inherent subjectivity of the diagnosis, based on the subjective interpretation of symptoms by both doctors and patients, leads to significant variations in diagnoses, even among experienced healthcare professionals. Additionally, the absence of specific tests contributes to the stigma and skepticism surrounding MCS, with some healthcare professionals reluctant to consider it a legitimate condition. This situation compromises the quality of care and exacerbates the challenges patients face in their medical journey.

2. Current approaches for diagnosing MCS:

To comprehensively diagnose MCS, a thorough clinical evaluation is essential, beginning with a detailed medical history and a meticulous analysis of symptoms and potential environmental exposures. Standardized questionnaires like the QEESI are used to assess the severity of symptoms and their correlation with chemical exposures. Laboratory tests and medical examinations, such as blood tests, allergy tests, medical imaging, and neurological and psychological evaluations, are required to rule out other medical conditions. Controlled provocation tests, although sometimes necessary to observe responses to specific substances, must be conducted with caution under strict medical supervision. A multidisciplinary approach involving allergists, immunologists, neurologists, psychiatrists, and psychologists allows for a holistic evaluation of MCS, integrating both physical and psychological aspects for an accurate diagnosis and effective management of the condition.

3. Potential advances and future research:

Research on chemical sensitivity is progressing through several strategic fronts. First, the identification of specific biomarkers is essential for developing more objective and reliable diagnostic tests, exploring genetic signatures, immunological markers, and distinct metabolic profiles. Simultaneously, the development of new diagnostic technologies such as advanced imaging, biofluid analyses, and immune response tests offers promising prospects for identifying MCS, provided they undergo rigorous clinical validations to ensure their effectiveness.

To improve patient management, it is crucial to enhance the education and awareness of healthcare professionals about chemical sensitivity, thereby reducing diagnostic subjectivity and promoting a consistent approach. Finally, promoting international collaboration among researchers, clinicians, and public health organizations is essential for developing standardized diagnostic criteria and innovative approaches. Research networks and international conferences play a central role in fostering this collaborative dynamic, which is conducive to significant advances in the understanding and management of MCS on a global scale.

The absence of specific tests for diagnosing chemical sensitivity complicates the task for both patients and healthcare professionals. By utilizing detailed clinical assessments, standardized questionnaires, exclusion tests, and a multidisciplinary approach, a more accurate diagnosis is possible. Research into biomarkers, diagnostic technologies, and improving healthcare professional training is crucial for enhancing patient care.

4.2 A Diagnosis of exclusion

The diagnosis of MCS often relies on a process of exclusion due to the absence of specific tests and the complexity of symptoms. This section provides a detailed examination of the concept of diagnosis by exclusion, its steps, challenges, and implications for patients.

1. Concept of diagnosis by exclusion:

Diagnosis by exclusion is a method used to identify a condition by eliminating all other possible causes of the symptoms presented by a patient. This approach is commonly used in cases where there is no definitive diagnostic test, as is the case with MCS. The goal is to ensure that the symptoms cannot be explained by any other disease before concluding a diagnosis of MCS.

2. Steps in the diagnosis by exclusion:

The diagnostic evaluation of MCS involves several essential steps. First, collecting a comprehensive medical history is crucial to examine past environmental exposures, family medical history, lifestyle habits, and psychological stressors that may influence symptoms. Next, a thorough physical examination is conducted to detect any clinical signs indicating another medical condition. This examination often includes the assessment of neurological, respiratory, dermatological, and cardiovascular functions. Laboratory tests, such as blood analyses, urine tests, evaluations of liver and kidney function, as well as medical imaging like MRIs or CT scans, are also performed to exclude underlying organic diseases such as metabolic disorders, chronic infections, autoimmune diseases, or cancers.

Skin or blood allergy tests are used to identify any potential allergies, while food intolerance tests help to exclude food-related reactions. Finally, prolonged monitoring of symptoms allows for observing their progression over time, their response to environmental changes or treatments, and a better understanding of potential triggers while ruling out temporary or reversible causes of MCS symptoms.

3. Challenges of diagnosis by exclusion:

The process of diagnosis by exclusion for chemical sensitivity is often complex and time-consuming for patients, who experience increasing frustration due to the quest for quick answers to their health issues. The multiple consultations and tests required are not only emotionally draining but also financially burdensome, as the costs of tests and consultations are rarely covered by health insurance. Additionally, the subjectivity in interpreting symptoms and test results leads to variations in diagnoses, with each doctor having their own interpretation, complicating the situation for patients seeking clarity. Furthermore, the lack of consensus and specific diagnostic criteria results in stigma and lack of recognition from some healthcare professionals, creating a climate of skepticism that hampers the quality of care and the necessary support for patients with MCS.

4. Implications for patients:

The diagnosis of MCS is often a complex and emotionally challenging process for patients. On one hand, the need for exclusionary diagnoses can lead to frustration and emotional distress, as patients face a lengthy wait for definitive answers and sometimes experience a lack of understanding from healthcare professionals regarding their condition. This situation can exacerbate existing psychological symptoms, such as anxiety and depression. On the other hand, the impact on quality of life is significant, with repeated consultations and invasive tests disrupting patients' ability to work, socialize, and lead a normal daily life. In this context, support from family, friends, healthcare professionals, and support groups plays a crucial role. An empathetic and understanding approach is essential to alleviate the distress associated with MCS and help patients navigate this challenging journey, providing the emotional support necessary to improve their quality of life.

The diagnosis of chemical sensitivity (complex and frustrating in the absence of specific tests) poses challenges for patients and healthcare professionals. Recognizing these challenges, improving diagnostic methods, and providing appropriate support are essential for better management.

4.3 Existing diagnostic criteria

Despite the absence of specific tests for diagnosing multiple chemical sensitivity, several diagnostic criteria have been proposed to assist clinicians in identifying this condition. Among the most recognized are the 1999 Consensus (Bartha et al.), the QEESI (Quick Environmental Exposure and Sensitivity Inventory), and the criteria developed by Dr. Claudia Miller. This section examines these criteria in detail, their application, and their advantages and limitations.

1. 1999 Consensus (Bartha et al.):

The 1999 Consensus, developed by Bartha et al., is one of the earliest efforts to establish standardized criteria for diagnosing MCS. This consensus was created by an international group of researchers and clinicians specializing in chemical sensitivity.

Criteria of the 1999 Consensus:

1. *Presence of recurrent and chronic symptoms:* Patients must exhibit recurrent and chronic symptoms related to specific environmental exposures.

2. *Multi-organ and multisystemic:* The symptoms must affect multiple organ systems, such as the nervous, respiratory, digestive, and integumentary systems.

3. *Low-dose triggers:* The symptoms must be triggered by exposure to low doses of chemical substances, well below levels considered dangerous for the general population.

4. *Partial or complete reversibility:* The symptoms should lessen or disappear when exposure to the triggers is eliminated or reduced.

5. *Absence of another medical explanation:* The symptoms should not be explained by another known medical condition.

Advantages and Limitations:

- *Advantages:* Provides a clear structure for clinical assessment. Widely recognized internationally by many experts.

- *Limitations:* May be too strict for some cases, excluding patients who could benefit from a diagnosis of MCS. Requires a thorough evaluation to rule out other conditions, which can be time-consuming and costly.

2. QEESI (Quick Environmental Exposure and Sensitivity Inventory):

The QEESI, developed by Dr. Claudia Miller, is a standardized assessment tool used to identify chemical sensitivities and evaluate their impact on patients' lives.

Components of the QEESI:

1. *Symptom scale:* Assesses the frequency and severity of common symptoms associated with MCS.

2. *Chemical exposure scale:* Measures the level of exposure to chemicals in the patient's environment.

3. *Sensitivity scale:* Identifies the patient's sensitivity to various chemicals, foods, medications, and other substances.

4. *Impact scale:* Evaluates the impact of chemical sensitivities on daily activities and the patient's quality of life.

Advantages and limitations:

- *Advantages:* Structured and easy-to-use tool for clinicians. Allows for a detailed assessment of exposures and symptoms.

- ➢ *Limitations:* Can be subjective, as it relies on patients' self-reports. Does not replace a comprehensive medical evaluation to rule out other conditions.

3. Criteria of Dr. Claudia Miller:

Dr. Claudia Miller, a recognized expert in the field of chemical sensitivities, proposed specific criteria for diagnosing MCS based on her research and clinical experience.

Criteria of Dr. Claudia Miller:

1. *Increased sensitivity to various chemicals:* Patients exhibit heightened sensitivity to a wide range of environmental chemicals.

2. *Identifiable triggers:* Patients can identify specific triggers for their symptoms, such as perfumes, solvents, pesticides, etc.

3. *Cross-reactivity:* Patients often show cross-reactivity to chemically similar substances.

4. *Impact on quality of life:* Symptoms and chemical sensitivities significantly affect patients' daily lives, limiting their activities and social participation.

Advantages and limitations:

- ➢ *Advantages:* Based on extensive clinical experience and detailed observations. Provides a practical approach for identifying MCS.

- ➢ *Limitations:* May lack formal standardization compared to other criteria. Partially relies on patients' self-reporting of symptoms, which can introduce subjectivity.

Diagnostic criteria for multiple chemical sensitivity, such as the 1999 Consensus, the QEESI Scale, and Dr. Claudia Miller's criteria, are valuable tools for clinicians. When used together, they provide a more comprehensive assessment of MCS. A multidisciplinary approach is essential for improving diagnosis and management of patients.

4.4 Assessing triggers

Assessing triggers is a crucial step in diagnosing MCS. It helps to understand the specific substances that provoke symptoms in the patient and to develop effective management strategies. This section explores the methods and tools used to identify and evaluate triggers, as well as the challenges associated with this process.

1. Methods for identifying triggers:

Evaluating chemical sensitivity relies on several methods and tools to precisely identify triggers and assess the impact of exposures on patients. First, a detailed history of environmental exposures is crucial, including cleaning products, cosmetics, perfumes, foods, medications, work and living environments, and leisure activities. Patients are encouraged to keep detailed logs of symptoms and daily exposures to establish meaningful correlations.

Elimination and reintroduction tests are also used, involving the sequential removal of suspected substances from the patient's environment to observe changes in symptoms, followed by their reintroduction to identify specific triggers. Environmental assessments are conducted by professionals to test air quality, analyze surfaces, and inspect building materials to identify potential sources of chemical substances.

Finally, controlled provocation tests are conducted in clinical environments under supervision, gradually exposing patients to suspected substances to observe reactions under strict medical monitoring. These integrated approaches are essential for an accurate diagnosis of MCS and for developing personalized management strategies aimed at minimizing symptoms and improving patients' quality of life.

2. Assessment tools and scales:

The assessment of MCS relies on various tools and methods to identify triggers and evaluate the impact of exposures. The QEESI (Quick Environmental Exposure and Sensitivity Inventory) is a crucial standardized tool that helps identify chemical sensitivities and assess how exposures affect the patient's daily life. Additionally, specific exposure questionnaires are used to gather details on the frequency, duration, and context of chemical exposures, which helps establish correlations between exposures and symptoms. Furthermore, environmental measurement tools such as VOC detectors, air quality monitors, and water testing kits provide objective data on the levels of chemical substances present in the patient's environment, facilitating the identification of potential sources of issues. These combined approaches enable a thorough and personalized assessment of MCS, essential for developing effective management strategies and improving patients' quality of life.

3. Challenges in assessing triggers:

Managing chemical sensitivity is complex due to several factors. First, patients may be exposed to a multitude of chemical substances in various environments (home, work, outdoors), making it challenging to identify specific triggers. Additionally, MCS symptoms may appear with a delay after exposure, complicating the establishment of direct links between exposure and reactions. Chemical interactions between different substances can also amplify reactions, further complicating the identification of individual triggers. The variability in individual responses to chemical substances requires a personalized approach for each patient. Moreover, psychological factors such as stress and anxiety influence symptoms, adding another layer of complexity to the assessment of triggers and overall management of the condition.

4. Strategies for managing identified triggers:

To manage chemical sensitivity, several strategies are essential. First, once triggers are identified, it is crucial to avoid these substances as much as possible by adapting cleaning products, cosmetics, and dietary habits, as well as making environmental modifications at home and work. Concurrently, improving indoor air quality through the use of air purifiers, regular ventilation, and selecting non-toxic building materials helps reduce exposure to volatile organic compounds (VOCs) and other irritants. In the workplace, specific accommodations such as fragrance-free zones, enhanced ventilation systems, and policies for using non-toxic products are implemented to protect patients. Education and awareness for patients and their families about potential triggers and avoidance strategies also play a crucial role in daily MCS management. Finally, regular medical follow-ups are necessary to monitor symptom progression, adjust management strategies, and provide ongoing support to patients.

Assessing triggers is crucial for diagnosing and managing chemical sensitivity. By using specific tools and questionnaires, clinicians can better identify the responsible substances and assist patients in adopting effective avoidance strategies. A thorough and proactive evaluation significantly enhances the quality of life for patients.

4.5 Obstacles to diagnosis

Obtaining a diagnosis of chemical sensitivity is often described by patients as a true obstacle course. This section examines the challenges patients face, the steps they need to undertake, and the specific difficulties associated with obtaining an accurate and recognized diagnosis.

1. Initial obstacles:

MCS presents several challenges due to its limited medical recognition by some healthcare professionals, often resulting in reluctance or misunderstanding of the symptoms reported by patients. The symptoms of chemical sensitivity are often varied and nonspecific, affecting different bodily systems, which complicates establishing a direct link to a specific chemical cause. Additionally, the lack of awareness and training among many doctors and healthcare professionals sometimes leads to misdiagnoses or incomplete diagnoses, thereby delaying appropriate management for patients with MCS.

2. Administrative and medical procedures:

Challenges associated with chemical sensitivity include the need for patients to consult a range of specialists, such as allergists, dermatologists, and neurologists, to find a competent professional in MCS. This complex diagnostic process also involves numerous repetitive tests and evaluations, often with different practitioners, which can be physically and emotionally exhausting, as well as financially burdensome. Additionally, patients must maintain comprehensive documentation of their symptoms, exposures, and medical history, requiring meticulous time management and organization to provide accurate information to healthcare professionals.

3. Financial challenges:

MCS imposes significant financial burdens on patients. On one hand, the costs of repeated consultations and tests required to establish a diagnosis of exclusion accumulate rapidly, often representing a substantial expense that is frequently not covered by insurance. Additionally, the inability to work due to symptoms and frequent medical obligations leads to a significant loss of income, exacerbating the financial stress experienced by patients dealing with this complex condition.

4. Personal and emotional challenges:

Patients facing chemical sensitivity often encounter complex challenges. On one hand, they must overcome skepticism and stigma from their surroundings and even some healthcare professionals, leading to social isolation and feelings of despair. Concurrently, the uncertainty involved in seeking a diagnosis and the associated frustration can lead to significant psychological distress, including anxiety and sometimes depression. Additionally, MCS has a profound impact on personal and family relationships, exacerbating tensions and misunderstandings as patients struggle to obtain an accurate diagnosis and manage their symptoms effectively.

5. Strategies to facilitate diagnosis:

To optimize the management of chemical sensitivity, several strategies are recommended. First, it is essential to identify and consult with specialists who are knowledgeable in MCS, which increases the likelihood of obtaining an accurate diagnosis and appropriate treatment. Simultaneously, actively participating in support groups provides not only emotional support but also practical advice and recommendations from experienced professionals. Comprehensive education on MCS, its potential triggers, and avoidance strategies is crucial; this involves researching reliable sources and sharing knowledge with healthcare providers for better individual management. Finally, maintaining systematic documentation in the form of symptom logs, exposure records, and medical consultations is essential for providing precise information to healthcare professionals. This helps in identifying specific patterns or triggers and allows for the appropriate adjustment of management strategies.

The diagnosis of chemical sensitivity is challenging, hindered by limited recognition, financial obstacles, and emotional distress. Despite these challenges, with perseverance, support, and a methodical approach, an accurate diagnosis is achievable. Raising awareness among healthcare professionals and improving the recognition of MCS are crucial for enhancing this process and supporting patients.

4.6 The role of specialists

Specialists play a crucial role in the diagnosis and management of MCS. Their expertise and experience are essential for evaluating symptoms, identifying triggers, and developing appropriate management strategies. This section explores the different types of specialists involved, their specific roles, and how they collaborate to provide integrated care to affected patients.

1. Types of specialists involved:

- *General practitioners and internists:* Often the first points of contact, they conduct an initial assessment of symptoms, rule out other common medical conditions, and refer patients to appropriate specialists.

- *Allergists and immunologists:* These specialists are essential for evaluating allergic reactions and immune sensitivities. They perform skin tests, blood tests, and other assessments to identify potential allergens.

- *Dermatologists:* Dermatologists examine skin symptoms related to MCS, such as rashes, redness, and contact dermatitis. They help identify environmental triggers that affect the skin.

- *Neurologists:* Neurologists assess neurological symptoms such as headaches, migraines, memory problems, and difficulties with concentration that may be associated with MCS.

- *Toxicologists:* Toxicologists specialize in studying the effects of chemical substances on the body. They help identify environmental toxins and advise on measures to reduce exposure.

- *Psychiatrists and psychologists:* Mental health professionals play a crucial role in supporting patients dealing with emotional distress and psychological disorders associated with MCS. They help manage anxiety, depression, and other psychological impacts.

- *Environmental medicine specialists:* These specialists focus on the interactions between human health and the environment. They assess environmental exposures and provide advice on risk reduction strategies.

2. Specific roles of specialists:

Specialists play a key role in the evaluation and diagnosis of chemical sensitivity syndrome. Allergists test for sensitivities to allergens, while neurologists assess neurological disorders. The tests include skin examinations, blood analyses, MRIs, and evaluations of air and water quality.

Based on the results, specialists develop personalized management plans, which include avoidance recommendations, medical treatments, and environmental adjustments. Regular follow-ups allow for the assessment and adaptation of treatments according to the patient's progress.

Coordination among specialists, often facilitated by general practitioners, is essential for integrated care of patients with MCS.

3. Support for patients:

Specialists play a crucial role in educating patients about MCS by providing clear information on potential triggers and management strategies. The goal is to help patients make informed decisions about their health. Additionally, they encourage patients to join support groups to share experiences and receive practical advice, while guiding them to appropriate community resources. On the emotional front, mental health professionals offer ongoing support to help patients cope with the psychological impact of MCS, aiming to improve their overall quality of life.

Specialists play a crucial role in the diagnosis and management of multiple chemical sensitivity. Their diverse expertise and a collaborative approach enable comprehensive and personalized care. Better coordination, integrated protocols, and ongoing support are essential for improving clinical outcomes and patients' quality of life.

4.7 Complementary assessment tools

The diagnosis of chemical sensitivity relies on a multidisciplinary approach and the use of various complementary assessment tools. These tools help to better understand symptoms, identify triggers, and develop personalized management strategies. This section outlines the key complementary assessment tools used by healthcare professionals in diagnosing MCS.

1. Questionnaires and assessment scales:

The QEESI (Quick Environmental Exposure and Sensitivity Inventory) is a crucial tool used to assess chemical sensitivity, covering sensitivities, environmental exposures, symptoms, and emotional reactions. It helps quantify the impact of MCS on patients' daily lives. Additionally, the Symptom Severity Score (SSS) is a scale used to measure symptom severity, track their progression, and evaluate the effectiveness of interventions. The Environmental Symptom Inventory (ESI) is another questionnaire that helps identify specific triggers and understand symptom patterns related to environmental exposures. These tools are essential for guiding the diagnosis and personalized management of MCS.

2. Controlled provocation tests:

Controlled environmental chamber provocation tests are essential for exposing patients to specific chemical substances in a regulated environment, allowing for the identification of immediate reactions and the determination of individual tolerance thresholds. Meanwhile, patch tests are primarily used to assess skin reactions by applying chemical substances directly to the patient's skin, helping to detect allergic or irritant responses.

3. Laboratory analyses:

Blood tests are crucial for identifying markers of inflammation, specific allergies, and other biochemical abnormalities associated with chemical sensitivity. They include analyses of IgE[7] levels, inflammation markers like CRP[8], and assessments of liver and kidney functions. Meanwhile, urine analyses are used to detect metabolites[9] of chemical substances and evaluate the body's ability to eliminate toxins, while also identifying recent exposures to certain chemical compounds in the patient's environment.

4. Environmental measurement tools:

The use of volatile organic compound (VOC) detectors is essential for measuring VOC levels in indoor air, substances often involved in chemical sensitivity reactions, thus identifying sources of indoor pollution. Meanwhile, air quality monitors play a crucial role in measuring various atmospheric pollutants such as fine particles, nitrogen

---

7 IgE (Immunoglobulin E) is a type of antibody involved in allergic reactions and defense against parasitic infections. It plays a key role in the immune response by binding to allergens and triggering the release of chemical mediators such as histamine.

8 CRP (C-reactive protein) is a protein produced by the liver in response to inflammation. It is used as a marker to detect and monitor inflammation and certain cardiovascular diseases.

9 Metabolites are intermediate or final products of metabolism, involved in biochemical processes necessary for maintaining life, such as energy production, growth, and cell repair.

dioxide, and carbon monoxide. This data is vital for assessing the patient's environment and recommending interventions to improve indoor air quality. Finally, mold tests are also important for detecting the presence of mold and other biological contaminants, helping to identify specific triggers of MCS in the patient's indoor environment.

5. Psychological assessments:

The use of the Beck[10] Depression Inventory (BDI) helps assess the level of depression in patients with chemical sensitivity, a condition often associated with significant psychological distress. This tool aids in providing appropriate psychological support by identifying depressive symptoms and guiding necessary therapeutic interventions. Meanwhile, the Hamilton[11] Anxiety Scale is used to measure the level of anxiety in patients, allowing for targeted psychological support and therapeutic interventions to manage anxiety associated with MCS.

6. Journals and symptom tracking:

Patients with chemical sensitivity are encouraged to use detailed journals to record their daily symptoms, potential exposures, and environmental conditions, which helps in identifying correlations between exposures and symptoms. Additionally, using dedicated mobile apps such as Symptomate, MyTherapy, CareClinic, Symptom Tracker, and Mood Tracker allows for real-time tracking of symptoms and exposures, facilitating systematic data

10 The Beck Depression Inventory (BDI) is a questionnaire used to assess the severity of depressive symptoms in individuals.

11 The Hamilton Anxiety Scale (HAM-A) is a clinical tool used to measure the severity of anxiety in patients.

collection and trend analysis for more effective management of the condition.

7. Holistic and complementary approaches:

Management of MCS benefits from integrative medicine consultations, which combine conventional and complementary approaches such as acupuncture, naturopathy[12], and personalized nutrition to effectively address symptoms. Practitioners can recommend therapies tailored to the individual needs of patients. Nutritional assessments conducted by dietitians are essential for identifying food sensitivities and proposing elimination diets that reduce symptoms. A balanced and tailored diet also helps to enhance resilience to toxic substances, thereby improving patients' quality of life.

Complementary assessment tools are essential for diagnosing and managing chemical sensitivity. By combining questionnaires, provocation tests, laboratory analyses, environmental measurements, psychological evaluations, and symptom tracking, healthcare professionals gain a comprehensive view of the triggers and impacts of MCS. This integrated approach enables the development of personalized management strategies and enhances the quality of life for patients.

4.8 Recommended Holistic Approach

The diagnosis and management of chemical sensitivity require a holistic approach that considers all physical, psychological, and environmental aspects of the condition. This section explores the key elements of a recommended holistic approach for

12 Naturopathy is a healthcare practice that uses natural methods to promote health and treat illnesses.

diagnosing MCS, aiming to provide comprehensive and integrated care for patients.

1. Understanding the holistic approach:

- *Definition of the holistic approach:* A holistic approach considers the whole person, including physical, emotional, mental, social, and environmental aspects of health.

- *Objectives of the holistic approach:*

  - Improve the quality of life for patients
  - Reduce the severity and frequency of symptoms
  - Promote overall well-being
  - Encourage self-management and empower patients

2. Comprehensive patient assessment:

- *Complete medical history:* Gathering a detailed medical history that includes symptoms, environmental exposures, family history, and comorbidities.

- *Lifestyle factors assessment:* Analysis of lifestyle habits such as diet, sleep, physical exercise, and stress levels.
- *Environmental assessment:* Inspection of the home and workplace environments to identify potential sources of chemical sensitivities.

- *Psychological assessment:* Examination of emotional and mental aspects, including stress, anxiety, depression, and coping[13] mechanisms.

---

13 Coping refers to the methods used to handle stress and challenges, including strategies to manage emotions and solve problems.

3. Multimodal interventions:

- *Conventional medicine:* Use of medications to manage acute and chronic symptoms, under the supervision of a qualified healthcare professional.

- *Complementary and alternative medicine:* Integration of complementary therapies such as acupuncture, naturopathy, and herbal medicine to support overall well-being.

- *Personalized nutrition:* Consultation with a nutritionist to develop a tailored diet plan, potentially including elimination diets to identify and avoid food sensitivities.

- *Stress management techniques:* Adoption of techniques such as meditation, yoga, deep breathing, and cognitive-behavioral therapy to manage stress and improve emotional resilience.

- *Environmental improvement:* Recommendations for enhancing indoor air quality, reducing exposure to household chemicals, and adopting eco-friendly practices.

4. Ongoing monitoring and support:

- *Regular consultations:* Ongoing follow-up with healthcare professionals to assess the effectiveness of interventions and adjust treatments based on the patient's progress and needs.

- *Support groups:* Participation in support groups to share experiences, receive practical advice, and benefit from emotional support.

1

- *Educational programs:* Educational programs to inform patients about MCS, management strategies, and the latest advancements in the field.

- *Online resources and technological tools:* Utilization of mobile apps, online forums, and other digital resources to facilitate self-management and symptom tracking.

5. Interdisciplinary collaboration:

- *Multidisciplinary care team:* Formation of care teams consisting of general practitioners, specialists, nutritionists, psychologists, toxicologists, and complementary medicine professionals.

- *Communication and coordination:* Encourage open and regular communication among care team members to ensure coordinated and integrated management.

- *Shared medical records:* Use of shared medical record systems to ensure real-time updates of relevant patient information and facilitate collaboration among healthcare professionals.

A holistic approach is essential for the effective diagnosis and management of Multiple Chemical Sensitivity. By considering all aspects of the patient's health, this approach enables the provision of integrated and personalized care, improves quality of life, and promotes overall well-being. Interdisciplinary collaboration, multimodal interventions, ongoing follow-up, and educational support are key elements in achieving the goals of this holistic approach.

Martin L. Pall

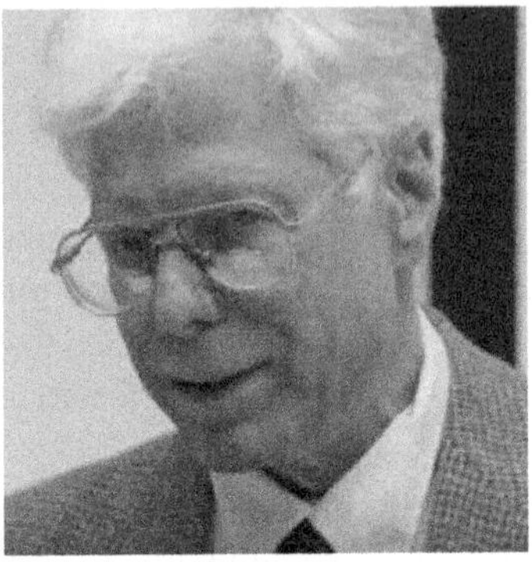

Martin L. Pall, an American biochemist and researcher, is known for his work on the molecular mechanisms of chronic diseases, including the effects of electromagnetic fields and chemicals on human health. His research has highlighted the role of free radicals and oxidative stress in conditions like Multiple Chemical Sensitivity. Pall proposed that excessive activation of the nervous and immune systems by chemicals and environmental stimuli could contribute to Chemical Sensitivity symptoms. His work has influenced the scientific and medical debate on MCS and inspired further research into its mechanisms and potential treatments.

Chapter 5
Living with restrictions

5.1 Creating a healthy home environment

For individuals with chemical sensitivity, a healthy home environment is crucial for minimizing symptoms and improving quality of life. Creating a safe living space free from chemical triggers requires careful attention to various aspects of the home, including air quality, the selection of materials and products used, and maintenance practices. This section explores the steps and strategies for establishing a healthy home environment for those affected.

1. Indoor air quality:

To maintain a healthier indoor environment, start by ensuring adequate ventilation using extractor fans in kitchens and bathrooms, and by regularly opening windows to promote fresh air circulation and reduce indoor pollutant buildup. Also, invest in air purifiers equipped with HEPA filters, which effectively remove fine particles, allergens, and volatile organic compounds (VOCs), and choose models that do not emit ozone. Finally, use indoor plants such as English ivy, areca palm, and spider plant, which are known to help purify the air by absorbing certain pollutants, thus improving the air quality in your home.

2. Selection of materials and products:

To create a healthier indoor environment, choose building and decorating materials with low VOC emissions, favoring eco-friendly and non-toxic paints, varnishes, and adhesives. Opt for furniture made from untreated solid wood or organic fabrics to avoid formaldehyde emissions from plywood or particleboard. Use natural and fragrance-free cleaning products such as vinegar, baking soda, and Castile soap, which are effective and non-toxic, thus contributing to a safe and health-conscious home environment.

3. Humidity and mold management:

To maintain a healthy indoor environment and prevent mold growth, keep indoor humidity levels between 30% and 50% by using dehumidifiers if necessary, especially in damp areas like basements and bathrooms. Regularly inspect your home for mold and remove it using natural solutions such as white vinegar or hydrogen peroxide-based cleaners as needed. Additionally, promptly repair any water leaks in roofs, walls, and plumbing to prevent moisture buildup and reduce the risk of mold proliferation.

4. Potable water supply:

To ensure optimal water quality at home, use high-quality water filters to effectively remove contaminants such as chlorine, heavy metals, and pesticides. Reverse osmosis[14] systems or activated carbon filters are recommended for their effectiveness. Be sure to regularly replace filter cartridges and follow the manufacturer's maintenance recommendations to ensure clean and safe drinking water for the whole family.

5. Pest control:

To maintain a safe and non-toxic home environment, prioritize natural pest control methods such as pheromone traps, organic essential oils to repel pests, and physical barriers to prevent their entry. Avoid using chemical pesticides indoors; if treatment is necessary, choose pest control services that employ non-toxic methods. This

---

14 Reverse osmosis filtration is a water purification process that uses a membrane to remove contaminants and produce clean water.

minimizes exposure to harmful chemicals while ensuring a safe environment for individuals sensitive to chemical substances.

6. Personal care products:

Opt for fragrance-free and hypoallergenic personal care products to avoid irritating chemicals found in synthetic fragrances, which is crucial for individuals with MCS. Also, use cosmetics and body care products made from natural and organic ingredients, carefully checking labels to avoid parabens, phthalates[15], and other chemical preservatives, in order to maintain a safe and suitable care routine for chemical sensitivities.

7. Education and awareness:

To maintain a safe environment for individuals with chemical sensitivities, start by educating all family members about the importance of practices aimed at avoiding harmful exposures. Also, inform guests and visitors about the measures in place to ensure safety, such as avoiding perfumes and chemically-treated clothing, and ask them to adhere to these practices when at your home. This collective awareness and effort contribute to creating a healthier and more supportive home environment for everyone.

Creating a healthy home environment is crucial for individuals with chemical sensitivities. By choosing non-toxic materials, controlling humidity and mold, ensuring clean drinking water, using natural pest control solutions, and opting for personal care products without irritating substances, you can significantly reduce MCS triggers. Educating family members and visitors

15 Phthalates are chemicals added to plastics to make them flexible and durable.

about these practices is essential to maintaining a safe and welcoming home environment.

5.2 Dietary challenges

Diet poses a significant challenge. Reactions to food additives, pesticides, and other chemicals present in foods can cause various unpleasant and debilitating symptoms. This section explores the specific challenges related to diet and offers strategies for managing and overcoming these obstacles.

1. Identification of food triggers:

To better manage food sensitivities, start by keeping a detailed food journal to identify foods and ingredients that trigger reactions. Additionally, under the supervision of a healthcare professional, consider an elimination diet where all potentially problematic foods are temporarily removed from your diet and then reintroduced one by one to identify specific triggers. Although controversial, some allergy and sensitivity tests can also provide useful insights into foods to avoid. Consult an allergist or nutritionist to determine appropriate tests and obtain a personalized management plan for your food sensitivities.

2. Food selection:

For a diet suited to chemical sensitivities, prioritize organic foods to avoid pesticides and chemicals used in conventional agriculture, which are often better tolerated. Choose fresh products such as fruits, vegetables, meats, and dairy, as processed foods often contain additives and preservatives that can trigger adverse reactions. Look for labels and certifications such as "no additives," "no preservatives," and "non-GMO" to select safer products, thereby minimizing exposure to harmful substances and promoting a healthier diet that respects individual sensitivities.

3. Meal preparation:

To maintain a safe diet suited to chemical sensitivities, prepare your meals at home to have complete control over the ingredients used, avoiding prepared foods and restaurant meals that may contain unlisted chemical substances. Use cooking utensils made from non-reactive materials such as stainless steel, enameled cast iron, and glass to prevent chemical contamination from kitchen equipment. Additionally, favor gentle cooking techniques like steaming, boiling, or low-temperature cooking to preserve nutrients and reduce the formation of potentially irritating compounds, ensuring safe and healthful food preparation.

4. Balanced diet and nutrition:

To maintain adequate nutrition despite a restrictive diet, consider carefully chosen dietary supplements, such as vitamins and minerals, to address potential deficiencies. Be sure to avoid chemical additives in these supplements. Introduce a variety of safe foods into your diet to prevent nutritional deficiencies and promote balanced nutrition. This diversification can also help identify new well-tolerated foods while supporting a healthy diet tailored to your specific needs.

5. Social and emotional challenges:

To manage the challenges of dietary restrictions outside the home, communicate your specific needs to hosts or restaurants and consider bringing your own safe meals or snacks. However, strictly adhering to these restrictions can sometimes lead to social isolation; therefore, join support groups or online communities to share strategies with others facing similar challenges. Additionally, managing stress associated with dietary challenges is essential: adopt techniques such as meditation, yoga, or therapy to cope with frustrations and anxieties that may arise.

6. Adapting eating habits:

- *Meal planning:* Plan your meals in advance to ensure a balanced diet and avoid last-minute food decisions that could lead to inadvertent exposure to triggers.

- *Flexibility and experimentation:* Be open to experimentation and the gradual introduction of new foods. Stay flexible and adaptive by adjusting your diet based on observed reactions.

- *Ongoing education:* Stay informed about new research and developments related to MCS and nutrition. Attend healthy cooking classes and workshops to learn new recipes and preparation techniques that are suitable for your dietary needs.

Food-related challenges are numerous and complex. Identifying food triggers, selecting safe foods, preparing suitable meals, and maintaining a balanced diet while managing social and emotional aspects are crucial for improving quality of life. With careful planning, professional guidance, and adequate support, it is possible to overcome these challenges and find viable solutions for a healthy and safe diet.

5.3 Dressing safely

Choosing clothing is crucial for avoiding skin and respiratory reactions. Textiles, dyes, and synthetic products used in clothing treatment can be potential triggers. This section explores the challenges and strategies for dressing safely, minimizing exposure to irritating substances.

1. Choosing materials:

When selecting clothing to minimize skin irritation, choose natural fibers such as organic cotton, linen, silk, and untreated wool. These materials are generally less irritating as they contain fewer synthetic chemicals. Avoid synthetic fibers like polyester, nylon, acrylic, and spandex, which can cause skin reactions due to their irritating chemicals. Also, look for eco-friendly certified clothing with labels such as GOTS (Global Organic Textile Standard) or OEKO-TEX Standard 100, which ensure the absence of harmful substances, providing a safer and more comfortable choice for sensitive individuals.

2. Treatment of new clothing:

To ensure safety, follow these steps when washing new clothing: start by washing all new clothes several times with a mild, fragrance-free detergent to remove chemical residues from the manufacturing process. Use hypoallergenic and organic detergents, avoiding fabric softeners and dryer sheets that contain irritating substances. To effectively remove chemicals, perform multiple rinses and consider using an extra rinse cycle. These precautions help reduce the risk of skin irritation and improve comfort for individuals sensitive to chemicals.

3. Clothing maintenance:

To minimize risks associated with chemical sensitivity related to clothing, follow these recommendations: Store your clothes in well-ventilated closets rather than plastic bags, which can trap chemicals and odors. Avoid dry cleaning, which uses persistent solvents; instead, choose water-based cleaning methods or look for eco-friendly dry cleaners that use natural solvents. For repairs or alterations, use natural threads and fabrics to avoid synthetic sewing products that may contain irritating chemicals.

4. Accessories and footwear:

Choose accessories made from natural materials such as untreated leather, wood, cotton, and linen, and avoid plastics and synthetic materials that contain irritating chemicals. Opt for shoes made from hypoallergenic materials and certified for sensitive skin, free from irritating chemicals. Regularly clean your accessories and footwear with natural cleaning products to prevent the buildup of dust and chemicals that could trigger reactions.

5. Adapting to climate and seasons:

Wear lightweight and breathable clothing in summer to avoid excessive sweating, which can reduce skin irritation. Materials like linen and lightweight cotton are well-suited for hot climates. In winter, opt for multiple layers of clothing made from natural fibers such as untreated wool and silk to maintain warmth without relying on synthetic materials. Also, use protective clothing like hats and gloves made from natural materials to effectively shield yourself from the sun and cold, minimizing the risk of skin reactions.

Dressing safely is a significant challenge for individuals with sensitivities. By choosing natural fibers, carefully treating new clothing, properly maintaining garments and accessories, and adapting to climatic conditions, it is possible to reduce the risk of reactions and enhance daily comfort. Ongoing education and awareness are also crucial for effectively navigating these clothing-related challenges and finding suitable solutions.

5.4 Cautious personal hygiene

For individuals with chemical sensitivities, personal hygiene products can often be a significant source of triggers. Many conventional products contain fragrances, preservatives, and synthetic substances that can cause skin, respiratory, and other reactions. This section explores the challenges and strategies for maintaining safe and effective personal hygiene while minimizing exposure to chemical irritants.

1. Choosing personal hygiene products:

Choose fragrance-free and hypoallergenic personal hygiene products, as synthetic fragrances are major irritants for individuals with sensitivities. Opt for products made from natural and organic ingredients, avoiding those containing parabens, phthalates, sulfates, and other chemical preservatives. Look for products certified by trusted labels such as COSMOS, Ecocert, and USDA Organic, which ensure the absence of harmful chemicals.

2. Daily hygiene:

Use gentle, plant-based soaps and cleansers free from chemical additives, such as Castile soap, or those made with oatmeal or honey. For shampoos and conditioners, opt for natural, sulfate-free, and fragrance-free options, and consider using baking soda or apple cider vinegar as alternatives. For moisturizers and lotions, choose those made with natural oils such as coconut oil, olive oil, and shea butter for effective hydration without chemical additives.

3. Oral care:

Use fluoride-free and fragrance-free toothpastes, and consider natural alternatives such as baking soda mixed with coconut oil for brushing. For mouthwash, choose natural solutions with ingredients like peppermint oil, tea tree oil, and apple cider vinegar, diluted in water for effective rinsing.

4. Feminine hygiene:

Use organic cotton, unbleached, and fragrance-free tampons and sanitary pads. For an eco-friendly alternative, consider medical-grade silicone menstrual cups or reusable organic cotton cloth pads. For intimate hygiene products, choose natural and fragrance-free options, and often prefer washing with plain water, which is less irritating than using chemical products.

5. Shaving and hair removal:

Opt for natural, fragrance-free shaving creams and aftershaves, such as those made with coconut oil or aloe vera, for a gentle and hydrating shave. For hair removal, choose gentle and natural methods like sugaring or beeswax waxing, which contain fewer irritating chemicals compared to traditional methods.

6. Deodorants:

Use natural deodorants free from aluminum and fragrance, favoring ingredients like baking soda, coconut oil, and essential oils for effective and non-irritating options. Embrace a certain level of perspiration as normal and healthy, changing clothes frequently if needed, and choosing natural fabrics that allow the skin to breathe.

7. Education and awareness:

Inform your healthcare and beauty providers about your chemical sensitivity, and request specific products that are suitable for your condition. Make a habit of carefully reading product labels to avoid potentially irritating ingredients, and familiarize yourself with the chemical names of substances to avoid. Share your experiences and tips with others who have MCS through support groups and online forums, where personal recommendations can be valuable for effective management of chemical sensitivity.

Maintaining careful personal hygiene is crucial for individuals with chemical sensitivities. By choosing natural hygiene products, avoiding fragrances and preservatives, and adopting gentle hygiene practices, it's possible to minimize reactions and maintain good daily hygiene. Continuous education and sharing experiences are also essential for navigating these challenges and finding suitable solutions.

5.5 Working in a controlled environment

The work environment presents a major challenge due to the potential exposure to various chemicals and irritants present in the air and office materials. Working in a controlled environment is crucial to minimize reactions and maintain optimal productivity. This section explores the strategies and adjustments needed to create and maintain a safe and controlled work environment.

1. Identifying potential triggers:

Identify the chemicals and irritants present in your workplace, such as cleaning products, adhesives, paints, construction materials, and office equipment. Assess indoor air quality by identifying pollution sources such as ventilation systems, printers, copiers, and fragrances. Keep a journal of your reactions to determine specific triggers in your work environment, which will help you adjust your strategies for managing multiple chemical sensitivities.

2. Communication with the employer:

Inform your employer about your chemical sensitivity and your specific needs related to this condition. Provide information on MCS and explain how it impacts your ability to work optimally. Make reasonable requests for accommodations such as using fragrance-free cleaning products, improving ventilation, or the possibility of working remotely if necessary. Also, provide appropriate medical documentation to support your accommodation requests and clarify the nature of your specific needs in the workplace.

3. Workspace arrangement:

Request a personal workspace or a private office if possible to better control your immediate environment and reduce exposure to triggers. Use hypoallergenic and chemical-free office equipment, such as untreated wooden furniture and accessories made from natural materials. Incorporate indoor plants like ivy, areca palm, and dracaena to improve air quality by filtering potential toxins present in your work environment.

4. Improving air quality:

Ensure that the workspace is well-ventilated by requesting your employer to check and maintain ventilation systems to ensure clean and adequate air circulation. Use air purifiers equipped with HEPA (High-Efficiency Particulate Air) filters to remove particles and pollutants from the air, which is especially beneficial in shared workspaces. Also, request a fragrance-free policy in the workplace to avoid potential triggers from cleaning products, personal deodorants, and air fresheners.

5. Adjusting work hours and arrangements:

Request flexible work hours to avoid times of high chemical concentrations, such as cleaning or maintenance hours. If possible, prioritize remote work to operate from a controlled home environment, significantly reducing exposure to triggers. Also, take regular breaks outside or in a safe environment to lessen continuous exposure to irritants and allow your body to recover effectively.

6. Personal management strategies:

- *Hand hygiene:* Use fragrance-free natural soaps for hand hygiene and avoid alcohol-based or fragranced hand sanitizers.

- *Hydration and nutrition:* Stay well-hydrated and maintain a balanced diet to support your health and resilience to irritants.

- *Relaxation techniques:* Practice relaxation methods such as deep breathing, meditation, or yoga to manage stress and enhance your resilience.

7. Training and raising awareness among colleagues:

Educate your colleagues about MCS, its symptoms, and its triggers to promote greater understanding and support. Also, encourage the implementation of office policies that favor fragrance-free products, improved air quality, and environmentally friendly cleaning practices. Finally, create a support network among your colleagues to share strategies, resources, and advice on managing MCS at work.

Working in a controlled environment is crucial for individuals. By identifying potential triggers, communicating with the employer, arranging the workspace, improving air quality, adjusting work hours, and adopting personal management strategies, it is possible to minimize reactions and maintain optimal productivity. Training and raising awareness among colleagues are also essential for creating a supportive and understanding work environment.

5.6 Limiting outdoor activities

Outdoor activities can be particularly challenging due to increased exposure to various pollutants, allergens, and irritants present in the environment. Limiting and managing these activities is essential to minimize reactions and maintain health. This section explores strategies and measures to safely participate in outdoor activities.

1. Identification of environmental risks:

Be aware of air pollution levels in your area, monitoring fine particles, exhaust gases, and industrial chemicals that may exacerbate MCS symptoms. Use apps and websites to daily monitor pollen levels and identify times of the year when they are highest. Be vigilant about the use of pesticides, herbicides, and other maintenance chemicals in public spaces like parks and gardens, as they can trigger reactions in sensitive individuals

2. Planning and preparation:

Select outdoor activities that minimize exposure to triggers by choosing less frequented locations away from main roads and industrial areas. Plan your outings during times when pollution and pollen levels are at their lowest, such as early in the morning or after rainfall, when the air is cleaner. Use filtering masks to protect your respiratory system, preferably those with fine particle filters like FFP2 N95 masks, which are particularly effective.

3. Clothing and accessories:

Wear covering clothing made from natural fibers to reduce contact with pollutants and allergens. Sunglasses can also protect your eyes from pollen. After being outdoors, immediately wash your clothes to remove pollutants and allergens, and take a shower to remove particles from your skin and hair. Carry a water bottle to stay hydrated and rinse your mouth or eyes if needed. Use fragrance-free wipes for a quick skin clean-up.

4. Management strategies during outings:

Limit the duration of your outdoor activities to reduce exposure to triggers and take frequent breaks in safe areas. Avoid high pollutant concentration zones, such as heavily trafficked roads, construction sites, and industrial areas. Stay well-hydrated and bring hypoallergenic snacks to avoid purchasing potentially problematic foods while outside."

5. Adapting activities:

Choose low-impact activities such as gentle walking, outdoor yoga, or reading in a park away from main roads to limit exposure to triggers. For sports and exercise, opt for indoor activities in controlled environments, such as gyms that use natural cleaning products. If you engage in gardening, create a personal garden using organic methods and avoid pesticides and herbicides to minimize the risk of exposure to chemicals.

6. Use of technology:

Use apps and websites such as AirVisual, BreezoMeter, and Air Matters to get real-time information on air quality and pollen levels. This will help you plan your outings by avoiding times of high pollution and pollen peaks. Also, check weather forecasts to avoid windy days, which can increase the dispersion of allergens. Keep your mobile phone handy to stay in contact with loved ones and to return home quickly if needed.

7. Awareness and advocacy:

Informing those around you about your needs and the risks associated with MCS is crucial for gaining their support and understanding. Join online or local support groups to exchange strategies and advice on managing outdoor activities. Also, participate in local initiatives to promote public policies that favor pesticide-free spaces and better air quality, thereby helping to create safer outdoor environments for everyone.

Limiting outdoor activities poses a major challenge for many individuals. By identifying environmental risks, planning outings carefully, wearing protective clothing, adopting management strategies during outings, and using technology, it is possible to reduce reactions and participate in outdoor activities safely. Awareness and community support are also essential for creating safer outdoor environments for everyone.

5.7 Traveling safely

Traveling presents significant challenges due to increased exposure to various irritants and pollutants. However, with careful preparation and appropriate strategies, it is possible to travel while minimizing health risks. This section explores the measures to take for safe travel.

1. Preparation before the trip:

Research your destination to identify risks related to air quality, seasonal allergens, and commonly used chemicals.

Carefully plan your itinerary by selecting transportation and accommodations with good environmental control. Consult your doctor before the trip to discuss preventive measures and obtain necessary prescriptions, such as antihistamines or inhalers. Create a checklist including medications, portable air purifiers, filtering masks, and fragrance-free personal hygiene products to ensure a safe and comfortable journey.

2. Choosing transportation:

- *Car:* If possible, travel by car to control your immediate environment. Ensure the car is well-ventilated and avoid air fresheners and other chemicals.

- *Plane:* Inform the airline of your specific needs in advance. Request seats away from restrooms and food service areas. Use filtering masks and bring fragrance-free wipes to clean your space.

- *Train and bus:* Choose transportation providers that allow you to control the environment as much as possible. Sit near windows for better ventilation.

3. Selecting accommodation:

- *Hotels and vacation rentals:* Look for accommodations that use eco-friendly and fragrance-free cleaning products. Call ahead to confirm their practices. Prefer lodgings with operable windows and individual ventilation systems.

- *Allergy-friendly rooms:* Some hotels offer allergy-friendly rooms. Inquire about these options and book in advance.

- *Portable air purifiers:* Bring a portable air purifier to use in your hotel room or vacation rental.

4. Food while traveling:

Opt for unprocessed and organic foods to avoid chemical additives and preservatives. Bring safe snacks that you have prepared yourself. Look for restaurants that use fresh, natural ingredients. Inform the staff of your dietary restrictions and request dishes prepared without chemical additives. Bring your own utensils and food containers to avoid cross-contamination and residues from cleaning products.

5. Managing exposure to chemicals:

Clean the surfaces of your accommodation upon arrival with fragrance-free wipes or a natural cleaning solution. Air out your room by opening windows as soon as possible to reduce the concentration of chemicals. Use portable water filters to ensure the water you consume is free from contaminants.

6. Strategies during the trip:

Practice relaxation techniques such as meditation, deep breathing, or yoga to manage stress, which can exacerbate MCS symptoms. Stay well-hydrated by drinking water regularly to maintain your immune system and reduce reactions. Ensure you get enough rest to allow your body to recover and remain resilient to irritants.

7. Awareness and advocacy:

Inform your travel companions about your needs and precautions to avoid chemicals and irritants. Join support groups to exchange travel tips for MCS; online forums provide valuable recommendations on safe destinations and accommodations. Participate in initiatives aimed at promoting safe travel practices and inclusive environments.

Traveling safely requires careful preparation, informed choices, and effective management strategies. By researching potential risks, selecting appropriate transportation and accommodations, taking food precautions, and using protective equipment, individuals can reduce risks and fully enjoy their travels. Awareness and community support are also essential to promote safer and more inclusive travel environments.

5.8 Maintaining social connections

Maintaining social connections is a challenge due to the need to avoid exposure to chemicals and irritants. However, preserving these relationships is essential for emotional and mental well-being. This section explores strategies and measures to maintain social relationships while managing MCS.

1. Open communication and education:

Informing your loved ones about your condition is essential to help them understand your needs and limitations related to MCS. Provide them with information on chemical sensitivity, its symptoms, and triggers through brochures, articles, or links to online resources to raise awareness and reduce misunderstandings. Engage in open and regular discussions with your loved ones to update your needs and adjust plans accordingly.

2. Adapting social activities:

Organize at-home activities to control the environment, such as movie nights, homemade meals, or board games, and invite your friends and family. Prefer outdoor outings in less crowded areas away from pollution sources, such as picnics in parks, nature walks, or visits to botanical gardens. Also, use technology to maintain social connections through video calls, online chats, and virtual games, thus avoiding exposure to triggers.

3. Arranging social environments:

Identify safe public spaces such as organic cafés and eco-friendly community areas that use fragrance-free cleaning products and ensure good ventilation. Ask your loved ones to avoid perfumes, scented personal care products, and recently dry-cleaned clothes when visiting to reduce triggers. When visiting friends or family, request preventive measures such as airing out rooms, using natural cleaners, and avoiding scented candles or incense to create an environment suited to your needs.

4. Participating in support groups:

Join local support groups to meet others living with Chemical Sensitivity and gain emotional support. Participate in online forums and discussion groups to exchange information, strategies, and encouragement. Get involved in collective activities suited for sensitive individuals, such as craft workshops, gentle yoga classes, or book clubs, to enrich your support network and enhance your well-being.

5. Strategies for special events:

For special events such as weddings, parties, or family gatherings, plan carefully in advance to anticipate potential triggers for your MCS. Discuss with the organizers to identify necessary adjustments, such as a quiet, well-ventilated area, ideally fragrance-free and with adequate ventilation. Opt for transportation options that minimize your exposure to irritants, such as traveling by personal car rather than public transportation, to maintain greater control over your environment during the journey.

6. Building new relationships:

Participate in events and activities tailored for individuals with MCS or that promote chemical-free lifestyles. Get involved in volunteering with organizations that share your values on health and the environment, which can expand your social network. Enroll in courses or workshops in controlled environments, such as natural cooking, art, or meditation, to enrich your social experience.

7. Emotional management and resilience:

Consult a therapist specialized in chronic conditions to manage the emotional stress of MCS. Use relaxation techniques such as meditation, mindfulness, or yoga to strengthen your emotional resilience. Engage in creative activities like writing, drawing, or music to express your feelings and reduce stress, thereby promoting increased emotional well-being.

To maintain social connections despite Multiple Chemical Sensitivity, open communication, creative adaptations, and proactive management of environments are essential. Inform your loved ones, adapt social activities, participate in support groups, and carefully plan special events to preserve meaningful relationships and an active social life. Emotional resilience and professional support are also crucial for addressing the challenges associated with MCS.

5.9 Isolation, a major risk

Isolation is a major risk due to the severe limitations imposed by the condition. Social isolation leads to negative effects on mental and physical health. This section examines the causes of isolation, its impacts, and strategies to prevent and overcome it.

1. Causes of isolation:

Avoiding chemical triggers creates involuntary isolation that limits social interactions and community activities. A lack of understanding from those around you can lead to feelings of judgment or misunderstanding, reinforcing social withdrawal. Chronic physical symptoms such as fatigue, headaches, and muscle pain also complicate participation in social activities. Additionally, physical and logistical constraints, such as difficulties with mobility and securing safe environments, actively discourage participation in social events.

2. Impacts of isolation:

Isolation significantly impacts mental health by exacerbating feelings of loneliness, depression, and anxiety, thereby affecting overall quality of life. Physically, it reduces social interactions and physical activity, which can lead to deteriorating health, including decreased mobility and weakened immune function. Additionally, isolation often deprives individuals of emotional and practical support from their surroundings, making it more challenging to manage their condition.

3. Strategies to prevent isolation:

Maintaining proactive communication with your loved ones is essential. Clearly explain your needs and find ways to stay connected, even from a distance, to preserve your social relationships despite the challenges posed by MCS. Utilize modern technology such as video calls, social media, and online forums for social interactions without the risk of exposure to triggers. Join local or online support groups specifically dedicated to individuals with MCS to share experiences, obtain advice, and benefit from emotional and practical support.

4. Creating safe social environments:

Creating safe spaces at home is essential for maintaining social interactions while minimizing chemical triggers. Invite your loved ones to your place, where you can control the environment to ensure your comfort and safety. Look for public venues that adopt chemical-free practices and request special accommodations if necessary for your well-being. For social events, consider outdoor meetings in parks or gardens, where the risk of exposure to chemicals is lower, facilitating your participation while preserving your health.

5. Adapted and alternative activities:

- *Creative hobbies:* Engage in creative and fulfilling activities that can be done at home, such as painting, writing, or playing music.

- *Gentle physical exercise:* Engage in gentle physical activities that can be done at home or in safe environments, such as yoga, tai chi, or stretching.

- *Community engagement:* Participate in community initiatives that are adapted to your needs, such as community gardening or online volunteering projects.

6. Professional support:

Consulting a therapist specializing in chronic conditions can help manage the emotions related to MCS and develop resilience strategies. Engaging a life coach facilitates setting realistic social goals despite restrictions. Participating in therapy groups provides regular social interaction and structured support, thereby enhancing coping skills in the face of MCS challenges.

7. Strengthening existing relationships:

Prioritize the quality of relationships by cultivating deep connections with individuals who understand and respect your specific needs. Engage in shared activities such as cooking, board games, or creative projects in controlled environments. Offer and seek mutual support to strengthen social bonds and enhance your self-esteem.

Isolation can be mitigated through proactive communication, the use of technology, the creation of safe social environments, and engagement in adapted activities. Professional support and the strengthening of existing relationships play a crucial role in this prevention. By adopting these strategies, individuals can maintain meaningful social connections, contributing to their overall well-being.

MCS

Chapter 6
Treatments for a better quality of life

6.1 Nutritional approach and supplements

An appropriate nutritional approach and the use of dietary supplements play a crucial role in managing chemical sensitivity. This section explores nutritional strategies, specific diets, and supplements that can help alleviate symptoms and improve quality of life.

1. Importance of nutrition in MCS:

A nutrient-rich diet can support the body's detoxification processes, particularly in the liver, which is essential for eliminating toxins. Foods high in essential vitamins and minerals can boost the immune system, helping the body better manage chemical exposures. Additionally, an anti-inflammatory diet can help reduce systemic inflammation, which is often present in individuals with chemical sensitivity.

2. Specific diets:

An anti-inflammatory diet can help reduce systemic inflammation by including antioxidant-rich foods such as berries and spinach, omega-3 fatty acids found in fatty fish and flaxseeds, and spices like turmeric and ginger. A hypoallergenic diet involves eliminating commonly allergenic foods such as gluten, dairy products, soy, eggs, and nuts, followed by gradual reintroduction to identify specific intolerances. The rotation diet, which varies the foods consumed daily, helps avoid cross-reactive food sensitivities and reduces the risk of developing new allergies. Additionally, a high-fiber diet based on vegetables, fruits, and whole grains supports intestinal health and promotes the elimination of toxins.

3. Foods to prioritize:

Cruciferous vegetables such as broccoli, Brussels sprouts, and cabbage support liver detoxification due to their specific compounds. Colorful fruits and vegetables are rich in antioxidants, protecting cells from oxidative damage. Whole grains and legumes, besides being fiber sources, provide essential nutrients that promote digestive health and stabilize blood sugar levels. Lean proteins like fish, poultry, and legumes are important for amino acids needed for cellular repair and immune function. Finally, healthy fats from avocados, nuts, seeds, and extra virgin olive oil support brain and cardiovascular health with their beneficial properties.

4. Foods to avoid:

Processed foods are often loaded with additives, preservatives, and artificial flavors, which can potentially trigger symptoms. Refined sugars can increase inflammation and disrupt blood sugar levels, affecting overall health. Caffeine and alcohol, by disrupting sleep and the nervous system, can exacerbate symptoms of certain conditions. It is also advisable to avoid food additives such as colorants, artificial flavors, monosodium glutamate (MSG), and sulfites to reduce the risk of adverse reactions.

5. Use of dietary supplements:

- *Essential vitamins and minerals:*

  Vitamin C: A powerful antioxidant that supports the immune system and detoxification.

  Vitamin D: Crucial for immune function and reducing inflammation.

Magnesium: Supports nerve and muscle function and helps reduce stress.

- *Antioxidants:*

Glutathione: A major antioxidant in liver detoxification.

Quercetin: An anti-inflammatory flavonoid that can help reduce allergic reactions.

- *Omega-3 fatty acids:*

Support brain and cardiovascular health, and have anti-inflammatory properties.

- *Probiotics:*

Promote a healthy gut microbiome, which is essential for digestion and the immune system.

- *Herbs and adaptogens:*

Turmeric: A natural anti-inflammatory.

Ashwagandha: An adaptogen[16] that helps manage stress.

6. Consultation with healthcare professionals:

Consulting a nutritionist or dietitian is essential for developing a personalized dietary plan that addresses specific needs and sensitivities. Physicians specializing in

16 Adaptogens are natural substances, such as ginseng and ashwagandha, that help the body adapt to stress and maintain balance.

integrative medicine can recommend appropriate dietary supplements and monitor their effectiveness and safety. Conducting food sensitivity tests helps identify intolerances and allergies, allowing for optimal customization of the diet.

A nutritional approach and the use of dietary supplements are powerful tools for improving the quality of life for individuals. By adopting specific diets, prioritizing certain foods while avoiding others, and incorporating appropriate supplements, it is possible to reduce symptoms, support detoxification, and strengthen the immune system. Consulting healthcare professionals is essential to personalize these approaches and ensure their effectiveness and safety.

6.2 Medical detoxification

Medical detoxification is a key approach. It aims to reduce the toxic burden in the body and enhance natural detoxification mechanisms. This section explores various methods of medical detoxification, their effectiveness, and the precautions to consider.

1. Principle of medical detoxification:

The primary goal of detoxification is to eliminate or reduce accumulated toxic substances in the body to decrease symptoms and improve overall health. Common methods include using medical treatments and supplements to support detoxification organs such as the liver, kidneys, intestines, and skin. These approaches aim to facilitate the effective removal of toxins and optimize essential bodily functions.

2. Types of medical detoxification:

- *Chelation*[17] *therapies* aim to remove heavy metals such as mercury, lead, and arsenic from the body. These therapies require close supervision by a qualified healthcare professional due to potential risks of electrolyte imbalance and renal toxicity associated with the treatments.

- *Liver support supplements:*

  Glutathione: A powerful antioxidant that plays a crucial role in liver detoxification.

  Silymarin (milk thistle extract): Protects liver cells and promotes liver regeneration.

  N-acetylcysteine (NAC): A precursor to glutathione that helps replenish its levels in the body.

- *Infrared sauna therapies* use heat to stimulate sweating, which facilitates the elimination of impurities through the skin. They are effective for dislodging harmful substances stored in adipose tissue. However, it is essential to stay hydrated and monitor body temperature to avoid heatstroke and excessive dehydration during these sessions.

- *Colon hydrotherapy* aims to cleanse the colon by removing accumulated waste and toxins, which can potentially improve digestive function and reduce the toxic load in the body. However, this procedure must be performed by a qualified professional to avoid risks of electrolyte imbalances and infections. It is essential

---

17 Chelation is a process where a substance binds to heavy metals to facilitate their removal from the body.

to follow specific recommendations and precautions to ensure the safety and effectiveness of the treatment.

3. Detoxification protocols;

- *Dr. Rea's Protocol:*

  Dr. Rea's protocol involves the use of supplements, specific dietary regimens, chelation therapies, and infrared saunas with the aim of detoxifying the body. This methodology is personalized to address individual needs and the specific types of toxins present in each patient, aiming to facilitate the removal of harmful substances and support overall health.

- *Step-by-Step Detoxification Protocol:*

  Phase 1: Preparing the Body by Enhancing Nutrition and Supporting Detoxification Organs.

  Phase 2: Active Detoxification with Chelation Treatments or Specific Supplements.

  Phase 3: Maintenance and Prevention with Lifestyle Modifications to Prevent Further Toxic Build-Up.

4. Precautions and Considerations:

When considering a detoxification program, it's essential to follow several important guidelines to ensure the safety and effectiveness of the process. First, always consult a physician or detoxification specialist to assess the specific risks and benefits for your situation. Second, tailor the treatment to your individual needs and overall health status to maximize benefits while minimizing risks. Third, maintain regular follow-ups with a healthcare professional to adjust the treatment based on your response and monitor progress. Fourth, ensure adequate hydration and essential nutrient intake to support the detoxification processes. Finally, be aware of potential side effects such as fatigue, headaches, and electrolyte imbalances, and consult a healthcare professional immediately if you experience severe symptoms. Adhering to these guidelines will help make your detoxification program safe and effective.

5. Complementary approaches:

When considering a detoxification program, several complementary approaches can be beneficial to support the process. Firstly, integrative medicine offers a holistic approach by combining conventional medicine with alternative therapies, which can optimize detoxification and promote overall body healing. Secondly, emotional and psychological support is crucial, as detoxification therapies can be emotionally challenging. Having support to manage stress and anxiety associated with this process is essential. Finally, moderate physical activity plays an important role by improving blood and lymphatic circulation, which helps in the elimination of toxins from the body. Incorporating these approaches can contribute to making your detoxification program more effective and beneficial for your overall health.

Medical detoxification is a crucial strategy for individuals with chemical sensitivity, aimed at reducing toxic load and improving quality of life. By following personalized protocols and taking necessary precautions, it is possible to support detoxification organs, eliminate toxic substances, and reduce symptoms. An integrative approach, well-supervised by healthcare professionals, is essential to ensure the effectiveness and safety of these treatments.

6.3 Nervous system regulation therapies

Nervous system regulation is essential. Nervous system regulation therapies aim to reduce stress, improve the body's response to environmental stimuli, and promote a better quality of life. This section explores various methods and techniques to balance and regulate the nervous system.

1. The importance of nervous system regulation in MCS:

Stress management is essential, as chronic exposure can worsen symptoms. By regulating the nervous system, it is possible to reduce this pressure and improve the body's overall resilience. Effective regulation can also increase tolerance to environmental triggers, thereby reducing the frequency and severity of reactions. Additionally, a balanced nervous system supports better digestion, optimal immune function, and contributes to improved mental health, thus providing overall health support for individuals.

2. Techniques for nervous system regulation:

- *Cognitive behavioral therapy (CBT)* aims to modify negative thoughts and behaviors associated with chemical reactions. It uses methods such as relaxation techniques, cognitive restructuring, and stress management exercises to help individuals better cope with symptoms and improve their quality of life.

- *Meditation and mindfulness* aim to reduce stress and increase awareness of the body and emotions. These practices include guided meditation, mindful breathing, and mindfulness exercises, which help cultivate present-moment awareness and improve emotional and mental well-being.

- *Biofeedback* uses devices to provide real-time information about physiological functions such as heart rate and muscle tension, allowing individuals to learn how to control them. This technique helps increase awareness of the body's responses and develop relaxation techniques, thereby promoting stress management and improving overall well-being.

- *Neurofeedback* aims to regulate brain activity using electroencephalographic (EEG) signals. This method relies on brain training based on real-time feedback, allowing for improved brain function and emotional regulation.

- *Yoga and relaxation exercises* aim to improve flexibility, reduce stress, and promote relaxation. Techniques include yoga postures (asanas[18]) to strengthen the body and enhance flexibility, breathing exercises (pranayama[19]) to calm the mind and boost vital energy, and deep relaxation practices such as yoga nidra to deeply relax both the body and mind.

3. Alternative and complementary therapies:

- *Acupuncture* aims to stimulate specific points on the body to balance the flow of energy (qi) and reduce stress. Its benefits include the ability to help alleviate physical and emotional symptoms associated with MCS, providing a complementary approach to enhance overall health and well-being for patients.

---

18 Asanas are yoga postures that improve flexibility, strength, and balance.

19 Pranayama is the practice of breath control in yoga, aimed at enhancing physical, mental, and spiritual health.

- *Craniosacral therapy*[20] aims to release tension in the craniosacral system to improve central nervous system function through gentle manipulations of the skull and spine.

- *Massage therapy*[21] aims to reduce muscle tension and stress using various techniques, such as Swedish massage, deep tissue massage, and muscle relaxation techniques.

- *Pulsed Electromagnetic Field (PEMF) therapy* aims to use electromagnetic fields to stimulate healing and reduce pain. This approach can offer benefits by enhancing cellular regeneration and reducing inflammation.

4. Adaptation and personalization of therapies:

Individual assessment is crucial in treating MCS, as each person reacts differently to therapies. It is essential to consult healthcare professionals to determine the most appropriate approaches based on each patient's specific needs. Combining different therapies offers synergistic benefits, such as integrating meditation with yoga or Cognitive Behavioral Therapy (CBT) with neurofeedback, which can enhance overall treatment outcomes. Regular follow-up and adjustment of therapies based on the patient's response are also essential to maximize benefits. This may

20 Craniosacral therapy is a gentle manual manipulation method aimed at assessing and improving the function of the craniosacral system, which includes the membranes and cerebrospinal fluid surrounding the brain and spinal cord.

21 Massage therapy involves using massage techniques to manipulate the muscles and soft tissues of the body, with the aim of relieving pain, reducing stress, improving circulation, and promoting overall well-being.

include using symptom journals, regular consultations, and collecting patient feedback to optimize treatment effectiveness.

5. Precautions and considerations:

Consulting qualified and experienced professionals in managing MCS and nervous system regulation therapies is crucial for effective treatment. It is recommended to seek certified practitioners with proven experience in treating patients to ensure appropriate care. Patients should also pay close attention to their bodies during therapies, noting any reactions or worsening of symptoms, and make adjustments accordingly with the help of their healthcare provider. Emotional support plays a critical role in managing the psychological impact of MCS and treatments. Resources such as support groups, group therapy, and individual consultations with psychologists or counselors can be beneficial in helping patients cope with the emotional challenges associated with their condition.

Nervous system regulation is a crucial component in the treatment of Multiple Chemical Sensitivity (MCS). By utilizing a variety of techniques and therapies, patients can reduce stress, improve their tolerance to environmental triggers, and enhance their overall resilience. A personalized approach, supported by qualified professionals, is necessary to maximize benefits and ensure patient safety. By combining these therapies with other detoxification treatments and nutritional support, it is possible to significantly improve quality of life.

6.4 Alternative and complementary medicines

Alternative and Complementary Medicines (ACM) play an important role in managing chemical sensitivity. These approaches offer various options to enhance quality of life, reduce symptoms, and support overall healing. This section explores different ACM practices and their application in treating Multiple Chemical Sensitivity.

1.Alternative and complementary medicine:

Alternative medicine refers to health approaches used in place of conventional medical treatments, while complementary medicine is used alongside conventional treatments. Their goals include reducing symptoms, improving the body's resilience to toxins, and promoting overall well-being and quality of life. These approaches aim to provide a range of therapeutic options to address the individual needs of patients.

2. Main alternative and complementary therapies:

- *Naturopathy* is based on using natural methods to support the body's healing capacity. Its principles include adopting personalized diets, using nutritional supplements, employing medicinal herbs, and applying stress management techniques. These approaches aim to enhance the body's natural healing mechanisms while promoting overall health and well-being.

- *Homeopathy* is based on the principle of similarity, often stated as "Similia similibus curentur" (like cures like), where substances that cause symptoms in a healthy person are used to treat similar symptoms in a sick person. This therapeutic approach uses highly diluted remedies, prepared according to specific methods, with the aim of stimulating the body's natural healing mechanisms.

- *Traditional chinese medicine (TCM)* encompasses various approaches such as acupuncture, Chinese herbal medicine, qigong[22], and Chinese dietary therapy. Its main goal is to balance Qi[23] (vital energy) and harmonize bodily functions to maintain health and treat diseases.

- *Ayurveda*[24] is a traditional Indian medicine system that aims to balance the doshas[25], or constitutional types, to maintain health and well-being. Its methods include the use of medicinal plants, a diet tailored to each dosha, therapeutic massages, and purification techniques such as Panchakarma[26].

- *Aromatherapy* aims to enhance physical and emotional health by using the properties of essential oils. Common applications include inhalation, diffusion into the air, massage, and therapeutic baths.

---

22 Qigong is a Chinese practice that combines movement, breathing, and meditation to enhance health and harmonize the body's energy.

23 The "Qi" in the word "Qigong" refers to the vital energy that flows through the body, which is essential for health and well-being in Traditional Chinese Medicine.

24 Ayurveda is a traditional Indian medicine system aimed at balancing the body and mind through diet, herbs, exercise, and wellness practices.

25 The doshas are the three fundamental energies (Vata, Pitta, Kapha) in Ayurvedic medicine that regulate the physiological and psychological functions of the body and mind.

26 Panchakarma is a series of purification and detoxification treatments in Ayurveda aimed at removing toxins from the body and restoring the balance of the doshas.

3. Benefits of ACM in MCS:

Alternative and Complementary Medicine (ACM) approaches can play a significant role in managing symptoms. They aim to alleviate manifestations such as headaches, fatigue, and digestive issues. Holistically, these methods support overall health by addressing both the body and mind. By personalizing treatments according to individual needs, they enhance their effectiveness and relevance for each affected person.

4. Considerations and precautions:

It is crucial to consult qualified and experienced professionals in alternative and complementary medicines (ACM) to ensure safe and effective treatments. ACM should be integrated with conventional medical care rather than replacing it, ensuring a comprehensive approach to healthcare. It is also essential to assess potential interactions between ACM and conventional medications to prevent adverse effects and optimize therapeutic outcomes.

5. Case studies and testimonials:

Clinical studies have demonstrated the effectiveness of alternative and complementary medicines in managing Multiple Chemical Sensitivity, including research on methods such as acupuncture, naturopathy, and homeopathy. These approaches have shown promising results in alleviating symptoms associated with MCS. Additionally, patient testimonials highlight the significant benefits of integrating ACM into their treatment, emphasizing notable improvements in quality of life through these complementary approaches.

6. Specific complementary practices:

- *Herbal medicine:* Utilization of specific medicinal plants to support detoxification and reduce inflammatory symptoms.

- *Breathing techniques:* Practices such as abdominal breathing and heart rate coherence to reduce stress and improve respiratory function.

Alternative and complementary medicines offer a range of valuable options. By integrating these therapies with conventional medical care, it is possible to enhance quality of life, reduce symptoms, and support overall healing. A personalized approach, supervised by qualified professionals, is essential to maximize the benefits of these practices.

6.5 Medication options

Medication options can play a crucial role in relieving symptoms and improving quality of life. This section explores various classes of medications used to treat symptoms, their effectiveness, and important considerations for their use.

1. Introduction to medication options:

The goals of treating Chemical Sensitivity include relieving acute and chronic symptoms, reducing inflammation and allergic reactions, and managing associated conditions such as anxiety and depression. It is crucial that medications used in the treatment be prescribed and monitored by qualified healthcare professionals, due to the complexity and specificity of the needs of MCS patients. Special attention should be given to avoid potential drug interactions and minimize unwanted side effects, ensuring a safe and effective therapeutic approach.

2. Commonly used classes of medications:

- *Antihistamines* are used to reduce allergic reactions and symptoms such as rashes, itching, and watery eyes. However, they can cause side effects such as drowsiness, dry mouth, and dizziness. It is important to monitor these effects while using these medications.

- *Corticosteroids* are used to reduce inflammation and immune reactions. However, they can cause side effects such as weight gain, hypertension, and immunosuppression. It is crucial to monitor these effects closely when using corticosteroids, especially over the long term.

- *Anxiolytics and antidepressants* are used to manage anxiety and depression associated with MCS. However, anxiolytics can lead to dependency, while antidepressants may cause side effects such as gastrointestinal disturbances, changes in appetite, and sleep issues. It is essential to monitor the use of these medications closely and work closely with healthcare professionals to adjust the treatment according to individual needs.

- *Anticonvulsants and mood stabilizers* are prescribed to manage neurological symptoms and improve emotional stability in individuals with MCS. However, these medications may have side effects such as drowsiness, dizziness, and weight gain. It is crucial to carefully follow medical recommendations and monitor any adverse effects throughout the treatment.

- *Bronchodilators and other respiratory medications* are used to relieve respiratory symptoms such as asthma and dyspnea in patients with MCS. They work by relaxing the muscles of the airways, making breathing easier. However, these medications can cause side effects such as palpitations, tremors, and headaches. It is crucial to follow medical guidelines for their use to minimize potential risks while optimizing their effectiveness.

3. Cautious and personalized use:

A thorough medical evaluation is essential for determining the appropriate medications and optimal doses in the treatment of Multiple Chemical Sensitivity (MCS). This process ensures that prescriptions are tailored to each patient's specific needs. Regular follow-up is also crucial for assessing the effectiveness of the treatment and adjusting prescriptions based on the patient's response, ensuring optimal symptom control. Finally, managing side effects is an integral part of medical monitoring, involving continuous surveillance and the implementation of strategies to minimize adverse effects and improve treatment tolerance.

4. Case studies and clinical outcomes:

Clinical studies provide concrete examples demonstrating the effectiveness of medications in managing symptoms of Multiple Chemical Sensitivity (MCS), highlighting outcomes achieved through various treatment protocols. At the same time, patient testimonials emphasize the positive impact of medications on their quality of life, detailing how these treatments have significantly reduced their symptoms and improved their overall well-being.

5. Integration with other treatments:

The multimodal approach in healthcare involves combining medication treatments with non-pharmacological therapies such as naturopathy, acupuncture, and cognitive-behavioral therapy (CBT). This approach aims to optimize therapeutic outcomes by considering the physical, psychological, and emotional aspects of patients. Care coordination, on the other hand, relies on collaboration among different healthcare professionals to ensure integrated and coherent management, thereby providing better oversight and appropriate follow-up of treatments.

6. Specific considerations for MCS:

Each patient has an individual response to medications, highlighting the crucial importance of personalizing treatments to optimize therapeutic outcomes and minimize side effects. It is essential to consider the long-term effects of medications, particularly those such as corticosteroids and anxiolytics, in order to make informed decisions about their prolonged use. Moreover, medications can often represent a less invasive alternative to medical procedures, thus providing an effective and better-tolerated therapeutic option for certain patients.

Medication options offer significant symptom relief for individuals. A cautious and personalized approach, supervised by qualified healthcare professionals, is essential to maximize benefits while minimizing risks. By integrating medication treatments with other therapeutic approaches, it is possible to enhance patients' quality of life and manage MCS symptoms more effectively.

6.6 Treatment of comorbidities

Individuals with MCS (Multiple Chemical Sensitivity) may have several medical and psychological comorbidities that require specific attention and appropriate treatment. This section explores common comorbidities associated with MCS and the treatment strategies that may be effective in improving patients' quality of life.

1. Common medical comorbidities:

- *Respiratory disorders* related to chemical sensitivity include conditions such as asthma, chronic bronchitis, and sensitivity to airborne pollutants. Recommended treatments include the use of bronchodilators, inhaled corticosteroids, and environmental allergen management techniques.

- *Dermatological* issues associated with MCS include skin reactions such as eczema, hives, and contact dermatitis. To treat these conditions, the use of antihistamines, soothing topical creams, and avoidance of skin triggers are recommended.

- *Gastrointestinal disorders* associated with chemical sensitivity include food sensitivities, irritable bowel syndrome (IBS), and gastroesophageal reflux disease (GERD). Recommended treatment includes dietary modifications, the use of probiotics, and medications such as proton pump inhibitors (PPIs) for GERD.

- *Neurological* issues related to MCS include chronic headaches, migraines, and cognitive disorders. Their treatment involves the use of analgesics, pain management therapies, and approaches aimed at improving cognitive function.

2. Psychological and emotional comorbidities:

- *Mood disorders* associated with chemical sensitivity include chronic stress, generalized anxiety, and depression. Recommended treatment includes psychotherapy, such as cognitive-behavioral therapy, the use of anxiolytic or antidepressant medications, as well as stress management techniques.

- *Sleep disorders* associated with MCS include insomnia, fragmented sleep, and sleep apnea. Recommended treatment includes the use of relaxation techniques, improving the sleep environment, and possibly the use of hypnotic medications under medical supervision.

3. Integrative approaches for the treatment of comorbidities:

A multidisciplinary approach is essential in managing MCS, involving collaboration among physicians, mental health specialists, nutritionists, and therapists to develop a comprehensive treatment plan tailored to each patient. Trigger management plays a crucial role, with precise identification and avoidance of environmental and dietary factors that may exacerbate comorbidities associated with MCS. Concurrently, an educational program is recommended for patients, aiming to inform them about symptom management and self-care, while providing ongoing support through support groups or social networks to enhance well-being and daily adaptation.

4. Individualized treatment strategies:

Each patient benefits from a thorough evaluation to identify the specific comorbidities associated with MCS, allowing for the creation of a personalized treatment plan tailored to their needs. Regular follow-up is essential to continuously monitor symptom progression, adjust the treatment based on the patient's response, and ensure effective management of their condition.

5. Impact on quality of life:

Effective treatment of comorbidities significantly enhances quality of life by reducing associated symptoms and increasing overall well-being. By managing these additional conditions effectively, patients are better equipped to handle the daily challenges associated with MCS, which reduces their overall burden and improves their ability to manage their condition optimally.

The treatment of medical, psychological, and emotional comorbidities is crucial in managing multiple chemical sensitivity. By adopting an integrative and individualized approach, it is possible to enhance patients' quality of life by reducing symptoms, minimizing complications, and promoting overall health. Careful monitoring and collaboration among various healthcare professionals are essential to optimize treatment outcomes and address the specific needs of each patient.

6.7 Essential multidisciplinary approach

MCS requires a holistic and multidisciplinary treatment approach to effectively address the complex needs of patients. This section explores the importance of collaboration among various healthcare and therapeutic professionals to enhance quality of life and manage symptoms.

1. Importance of the multidisciplinary approach:

Healthcare professionals from various specialties contribute to a comprehensive understanding of the underlying mechanisms of MCS and its impacts on physical and mental health. Each professional brings unique expertise to address the specific medical, psychological, and emotional symptoms associated with MCS. A multidisciplinary approach allows for the development of an individualized treatment plan that takes into account the unique needs of each patient and their responses to different therapeutic modalities.

2. Professionals engaged in a multidisciplinary approach:

- *General practitioners and specialists:* Initial assessment, diagnosis, and management of specific medical symptoms such as respiratory, dermatological, and gastrointestinal disorders.

- *Allergists and immunologists:* Identification of allergens and sensitivities, management of exacerbated immune responses, and development of avoidance strategies.

- *Psychiatrists and psychologists:* Assessment and treatment of anxiety disorders, depression, and post-traumatic stress often associated with CFS.

- *Nutritionists and dietitians:* Development of specific diets to minimize food triggers and support digestive and immune health.

- *Physical therapists and occupational therapists:* Customized exercise and physical rehabilitation programs to improve functionality and overall quality of life.

- *Complementary and alternative medicine (CAM) practitioners:* Use of techniques such as acupuncture, chiropractic[27] care, and homeopathy to complement conventional medical approaches.

3. Care coordination and communication:

Multidisciplinary case meetings involve regular discussions among care team members to review patient progress, adjust the treatment plan, and explore new approaches. Informed consent requires actively involving the patient in decisions about their treatment plan, considering their personal preferences and health goals. Continuous follow-up is crucial for assessing the effectiveness of the treatment, monitoring side effects, and adjusting interventions based on the patient's evolving condition.

4. Advantages of a multidisciplinary approach:

Optimizing outcomes for patients with sensitivity syndrome involves maximizing the chances of success by combining different perspectives and therapeutic modalities tailored to their varied needs. Reducing complications aims to minimize adverse medical and psychological effects through proactive and coordinated management of symptoms and comorbidities. Finally, improving quality of life involves a comprehensive approach that thoroughly addresses the multiple aspects of the condition, thus supporting patients' physical and emotional well-being.

A multidisciplinary approach is crucial for effectively treating chemical sensitivity. Integrating diverse healthcare professionals' expertise improves symptom management, reduces complications, and optimizes patients' quality of life.

27 Chiropractic care is a healthcare practice focused on the diagnosis and treatment of musculoskeletal disorders, particularly those of the spine, through manual manipulations and adjustments.

Close collaboration and coordinated care are essential for achieving lasting positive outcomes.

6.8 The importance of self-management

MCS requires not only appropriate medical and therapeutic treatments but also an active self-management approach by patients. This section explores the importance of self-management in the daily management of MCS and practical strategies to help patients take control of their health and well-being.

1. Understanding self-management:

Self-management refers to the actions taken by individuals to promote their health, manage their symptoms, and improve their quality of life. This involves encouraging patients to play an active role in their treatment and make informed health decisions, thereby fostering empowerment[28].

2. Self-management strategies for MCS:

Educating oneself about chemical sensitivity involves understanding its triggers and health impacts to avoid harmful exposures. Managing environmental triggers includes reducing exposure to chemicals and allergens by modifying home and work environments. Adopting a healthy lifestyle with a balanced diet, regular exercise, and stress management strengthens the immune system. Relaxation techniques like meditation, yoga, and deep breathing reduce stress reactions. Keeping a symptom journal helps track triggers, symptoms, and treatment

28 Empowerment enables individuals to take control of their lives by acquiring skills, confidence, and resources to achieve their goals and influence their environment.

responses to adjust self-management strategies. Open communication with the healthcare team is essential for sharing progress, discussing concerns, and adjusting the treatment plan.

3. Challenges and adaptations:

Individual responses to self-management strategies vary from patient to patient; therefore, it is crucial to explore and adapt different approaches to find what works best for each individual. Social and community support plays an important role: seeking support from family, friends, and MCS patient support groups allows for sharing experiences, obtaining advice, and feeling supported in the journey of managing the condition.

4. Integration into daily life:

Establishing a structured routine includes creating a consistent daily schedule to enhance well-being and minimize trigger exposure. For professional adaptations, it's essential to work with employers to implement adjustments that reduce health risks and support effective MCS management.

Self-management is a crucial pillar in the effective management of chemical sensitivity. By adopting appropriate self-management strategies, patients can not only reduce MCS symptoms but also enhance their overall quality of life. Education, informed decision-making, and collaboration with a multidisciplinary care team are key elements in supporting effective and sustainable self-management of MCS.

Claudia S. Miller

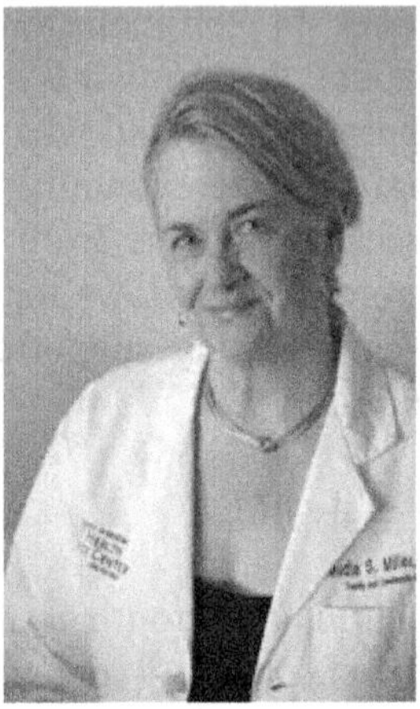

Claudia S. Miller is a renowned American physician and researcher in environmental medicine. She is known for her work on multiple chemical sensitivities and central sensitivity syndrome (CSS), conditions where patients have excessive reactions to low levels of chemicals and other environmental factors. Miller is a professor emerita at the University of Texas at San Antonio (UT Health San Antonio) and developed the "toxicant-induced loss of tolerance" (TILT) model, a theory explaining how chemical exposures can lead to a loss of tolerance in some individuals. Her research has significantly contributed to the understanding of the impacts of the environment on human health.

Chapter 7
Resources and appendices

7.1 List of resources and organizations

For individuals with multiple chemical sensitivity (MCS) or not, it is crucial to have access to appropriate resources and support. Here is a list of associations and useful information for patients and healthcare professionals:

- *FRANCE MCS European Associative Collective of Multiple Chemical Sensitivity Syndrome:* The Collective is a French organization that represents the interests of people suffering from Multiple Chemical Sensitivity Syndrome. Its goal is to raise public awareness, support patients, promote research, and defend the rights of affected individuals in Europe.
  Website: *francemcs.com*

- *National Multiple Chemical Sensitivity Foundation (NMCSF):* Research, education, and support for people with MCS.
  Website: *http://ehnca.org*

- *International Society for Environmentally Acquired Illnesses (ISEAI):* International research and support for people affected by diseases.
  Website: *https://iseai.org*

- *The Environmental Medicine Foundation (EMF):* Research and support for people affected by environmental illnesses, including chemical sensitivity. (Although this organization has international links, it is also active in the United Kingdom.)
  Website:
  https://www.environmentalmedicinefoundation.org

- *The British Society for Environmental Medicine (BSEM):* Education, research, and support in environmental medicine, including chemical sensitivity.
  Website: *https://bsem.org.uk*

- *Allergy and Environmental Sensitivity Support and Research Association (AESSRA):* Support for people with chemical and environmental sensitivities, as well as the promotion of research and education in this field.
  Website: *https://aessra.org*

- *Emerge Australia:* Although primarily focused on Chronic Fatigue Syndrome/Myalgic Encephalomyelitis, this organization also supports individuals with MCS and other environmental sensitivities.
  Website: *https://www.emerge.org.au*

- *MCS-Aware Australia:* Raising awareness, support, and education for individuals with MCS and other environmental illnesses.
  Website: *https://mcs-aware.org*

- *Chemical Sensitivity Foundation (CSF):* Organization providing information on chemical sensitivity, current research, and advice for daily management.
  Website: *www.chemicalsensitivityfoundation.org*

- *ASEQ-EHAQ L'Association pour la santé environnementale du Québec / Environmental Health Association of Québec:* It supports individuals affected by environmental health issues, such as MCS, by providing resources, information, and promoting recognition of these conditions.
  Website: *https://aseq-ehaq.ca*

The list of resources and organizations provides easy access to information, community support, and research networks on

MCS. It plays a crucial role in education, advocacy, and support for affected individuals, thereby enhancing disease management and quality of life.

7.2 Recommended readings

To deepen your understanding of MCS and explore various perspectives on managing this condition, here is a selection of recommended readings:

1. Specialized books:

- *Chemical Exposures: Low Levels and High Stakes* by Nicholas A. Ashford and Claudia S. Miller.

- *Multiple Chemical Sensitivities: A Survival Guide* by Pamela Reed Gibson.

- *La Sensibilité Chimique Multiple M.C.S. "Au-delà du Combat Quotidien":* Discover how it can affect you through this guide to understanding and managing difficulties by Marc Sachot.

2. Articles and Clinical Studies:

- *PubMed* is a free database, primarily from the National Library of Medicine in the United States, providing access to millions of abstracts and research articles in the fields of medicine and life sciences.

3. Online resources:

- *Environmental Health Trust (EHT):* Offers articles and resources on environmental exposures and health.

- *Planet Thrive:* Provides publications and guides on chemical sensitivity and its implications.

4. Specialized journals:

- *Journal of Occupational and Environmental Medicine:* Includes articles on the effects of chemical and environmental exposures on health.

The recommended readings provide essential information on MCS, including its mechanisms, health impacts, and best practices for management. They are crucial for patients, healthcare professionals, and researchers to enhance understanding of this complex condition and to effectively support those affected by it.

7.3 Environmental pathology centers

- **Environmental Health Center (**Dallas, Texas**)**
  Founded by Dr. William J. Rea in 1984, the center has become a leader in the field of environmental medicine, particularly in the diagnosis and treatment of chemical sensitivity disorders and environmental diseases.

- **The Cleveland Clinic** (Cleveland, Ohio)
  Cleveland Clinic offers services for environmental-related disorders, with specialists who can address issues of chemical sensitivity.

- **Johns Hopkins Medicine** (Baltimore, Maryland)
  Johns Hopkins offers consultations and research on environmental diseases, including disorders related to chemical sensitivity.

- **University of California, San Francisco (UCSF) Medical Center** (San Francisco, California)
  UCSF offers specialized care for environmental diseases and can provide evaluations for symptoms of chemical sensitivity.

- **Mayo Clinic** (Rochester, Minnesota)
  Mayo Clinic is renowned for its comprehensive care and can provide evaluations for chemical sensitivity as part of environmental disorders.

- **Breakspear Medical Clinic**
  (Hemel Hempstead,Hertfordshire, England)
  Breakspear is a clinic specializing in the diagnosis and treatment of environmental disorders, including multiple chemical sensitivity (MCS).

MCS

Anne Steinemann

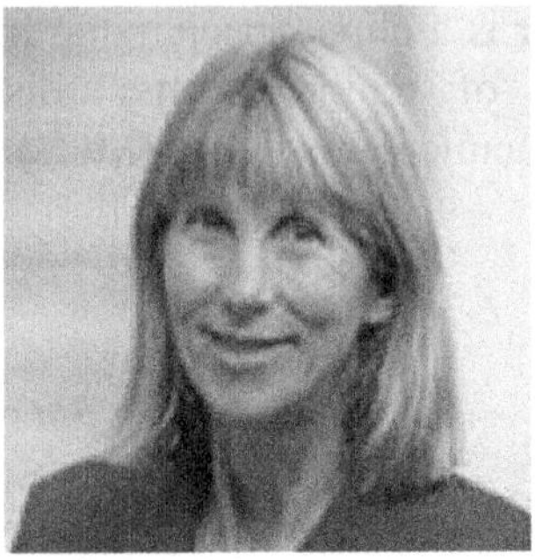

Anne Steinemann, an American environmental engineer and researcher, specializes in indoor air quality and the health impacts of fragrances. Holding a Ph.D. from Stanford University, she has taught at the University of Washington and the University of Melbourne. Her research frequently uncovers unlabeled volatile organic compounds (VOCs) in everyday consumer products. Steinemann advocates for greater transparency in labeling and raises public awareness about the risks of synthetic fragrances. Her work influences chemical safety policies to promote safer indoor environments.

Conclusion

Multiple chemical sensitivity (MCS) represents a significant challenge for those who suffer from it, profoundly affecting their quality of life and their ability to live in an everyday environment often filled with common yet potentially harmful substances. Throughout this book, we have explored various aspects of MCS, from its symptoms and management methods to diagnostic challenges and impacts on patients' daily lives.

It is crucial to emphasize the importance of increased recognition of MCS by the medical community. Too often, patients encounter a lack of understanding from healthcare professionals, leading to misdiagnoses or inappropriate treatments. By educating doctors and specialists about the unique characteristics of chemical sensitivity, we can significantly improve outcomes for patients by providing more effective and targeted support.

Moreover, it is essential to encourage further research on MCS. While progress has been made in recognizing this condition, much remains to be discovered about its underlying mechanisms, specific triggers, and the most effective therapeutic approaches. Investments in research can lead to new treatment strategies and more personalized management recommendations, thereby addressing the diverse needs of affected patients.

Finally, let us call for more compassion towards patients with MCS. Living with an exacerbated sensitivity to chemicals leads to social isolation, professional difficulties, and significant emotional challenges. By acknowledging and validating their experiences, we can help create a more supportive and inclusive environment for everyone living with this complex condition.

In conclusion, by enhancing recognition, advancing research, and demonstrating increased compassion toward patients, we can significantly improve the quality of life for individuals with MCS. This is a call to action for all stakeholders involved in healthcare and beyond, to advance our understanding and support for these often overlooked yet resilient individuals.

MCS

Biblical references

Here is a list of books on chemical sensitivity, written by doctors, that served as references for writing this book:

Dr. Theron Randolph was a pioneer in the field of environmental medicine and multiple chemical sensitivity (MCS). Here are some of his important books:

- *"An Alternative Approach to Allergies: The New Field of Clinical Ecology Unravels the Environmental Causes of Mental and Physical Ills":* This book presents Dr. Randolph's alternative approach to understanding and treating allergies and environmental illnesses, with a focus on the environmental causes of mental and physical diseases.

- *"Human Ecology and Susceptibility to the Chemical Environment":* A work that explores the relationship between human ecology and susceptibility to environmental chemical substances, based on Dr. Randolph's research and clinical experience.

- *"Environmental Medicine: Beginnings and Bibliographies of Clinical Ecology":* This book addresses the beginnings and bibliographies of clinical ecology, providing a valuable reference for those interested in the history and development of this medical field.

These books are essential references for environmental medicine, clinical ecology, and chemical sensitivity. Dr. Theron Randolph played a crucial role in promoting the environmental approach for diagnosing and managing complex health conditions, influencing many clinicians and researchers.

William J. Rea, a pioneering physician in the field of environmental medicine and multiple chemical sensitivity, has written several important books. Here is a list of books authored by William J. Rea:

➢ *"Chemical Sensitivity, Volume I: Principles and Mechanisms":* This book explores the principles and underlying mechanisms of chemical sensitivity, offering an in-depth overview based on Rea's research and clinical experience.

➢ *"Chemical Sensitivity, Volume II: Sources of Total Body Load":* The second volume of the series addresses sources of total body burden from chemicals and their impact on health.

➢ *"Chemical Sensitivity, Volume III: Clinical Manifestations of Pollutant Overload":* This book focuses on the clinical manifestations of pollutant overload, providing valuable information for clinicians and researchers.

➢ *"Chemical Sensitivity: Tools, Diagnosis and Method of Treatment" Volume IV:* A work that explores diagnostic tools and treatment methods for chemical sensitivity and other environmental illnesses.

➢ *"Reversibility of Chronic Degenerative Disease and Hypersensitivity, Volume 1: Regulating Mechanisms of Chemical Sensitivity":* In this book, Rea examines the regulatory mechanisms of chemical sensitivity and explores the reversibility of chronic degenerative diseases.

➢ *"Reversibility of Chronic Degenerative Disease and Hypersensitivity, Volume 2: The Clinical Manifestations of Chemical Sensitivity":* The second volume of this series examines the clinical manifestations of chemical sensitivity and offers treatment strategies based on the principles of environmental medicine.

These works are widely recognized in the field of environmental medicine and chemical sensitivity for their contribution to understanding underlying mechanisms, diagnostics, and treatment approaches. They are intended for both healthcare professionals and patients seeking to deepen their understanding of this complex condition.

Claudia S. Miller, a renowned expert in environmental health and multiple chemical sensitivity, has written several important books. Here is one of the significant books authored by Claudia S. Miller:

- *"Chemical Exposures: Low Levels and High Stakes":* Co-écrit avec Nicholas A. Ashford: This book explores the impacts of low-level chemical exposure on human health, including multiple chemical sensitivity (MCS).

Claudia S. Miller is also the author of numerous research articles and book chapters that address various aspects of environmental health, including MCS. Her work is widely recognized for its contribution to understanding the impacts of environmental exposures on human health.

Martin L. Pall is a renowned researcher in the field of biomedical sciences, primarily known for his research on the biochemical mechanisms involved in various conditions of chemical and electromagnetic sensitivity. Here is a book by Martin L. Pall:

- *"Explaining 'Unexplained Illnesses': Disease Paradigm for Chronic Fatigue Syndrome, Multiple Chemical Sensitivity, Fibromyalgia, Post-Traumatic Stress Disorder, Gulf War Syndrome and Others":* This book explores chronic diseases such as chronic fatigue syndrome, multiple chemical sensitivity, fibromyalgia, Gulf War syndrome, and others, proposing a new paradigm to explain them.

Martin L. Pall has authored numerous research articles in specialized scientific journals, exploring the molecular mechanisms of stress-related diseases, including chemical and electromagnetic sensitivity. He is widely respected for his scientific contributions in the field of environmental health, particularly for his work on the complex biochemical mechanisms underlying physiological responses to environmental stresses. His writings are essential for those seeking to deepen their understanding of diseases related to chemical and electromagnetic sensitivity.

Sherry A. Rogers is a physician and prolific author in the field of environmental health and integrative medicine. Here are some of her important books:

- *"Detoxify or Die":* This book examines the importance of detoxification to counteract the effects of toxic environmental chemicals and proposes effective detoxification strategies.

- *"No More Heartburn: Stop the Pain in 30 Days--Naturally!: The Safe, Effective Way to Prevent and Heal Chronic Gastrointestinal Disorders":* Although focused on gastrointestinal disorders, this book offers insights into the natural approach for treating chronic diseases, considering environmental factors.

- *"Tired or Toxic?: A Blueprint for Health":* A guide that examines how environmental toxicity can affect overall health and offers solutions for improving health by eliminating toxins.

Sherry A. Rogers is recognized for her innovative approaches in environmental medicine, highlighting the importance of the environment on human health and offering practical solutions for the prevention and treatment of diseases related to chemical sensitivity and other environmental factors.

Pamela Reed Gibson is a recognized researcher and author in the field of multiple chemical sensitivity (MCS) and environmental illnesses. Here is one of her important books:

- *"Multiple Chemical Sensitivity: A Survival Guide":* This book is a practical guide for understanding and managing multiple chemical sensitivity, offering helpful advice for patients and their families.

Pamela Reed Gibson is also the author of numerous research articles and book chapters that deepen the scientific understanding of MCS and associated environmental illnesses. Her contributions are significant for those seeking to better understand and manage this complex condition.

Dr. Anne Steinemann is a renowned researcher and author in the field of chemicals and environmental health. Here is one of her books:

- *"Exposure Analysis":* This book analyzes exposures and is the first comprehensive resource on environmental pollutants and their impacts on human health. It explores exposure to volatile organic compounds, particulate matter, pesticides, dioxane (a solvent), dust, and secondhand smoke, while also addressing personal monitors, mathematical modeling, biomarkers, laws and policies, as well as inhalation, ingestion, and skin exposure pathways. It offers concepts and analytical methods for identifying pollution sources, understanding causes, measuring exposures, and developing public health strategies.

Anne Steinemann has written numerous research articles in specialized scientific journals, examining the effects of chemicals on human health and strategies to minimize exposure. She is recognized for her work on chemicals and their impact on human health, making her a key voice in the field of environmental health and chemical risk management in our daily lives.

Dr. Jeffery A. Molot is a Canadian physician specializing in the treatment of multiple chemical sensitivity and environmental illnesses. Here is one of his books:

- *"12,000 Canaries Can't Be Wrong: What's Making You Sick and What You Can Do About It":* This book examines the causes and treatments of environmental illnesses, including MCS, based on Dr. Molot's clinical experience and case studies.

Dr. Molot has written and contributed to several research articles in medical and scientific journals, exploring the clinical and therapeutic aspects of environmental diseases. He is also recognized for his numerous presentations at medical and environmental conferences, sharing his expertise on MCS and other conditions related to environmental exposure. These resources are valuable for those seeking to understand the medical and scientific aspects of chemical sensitivity and to explore treatment and management options for this complex condition.

Dr. Jean Monro is a British physician specializing in the treatment of environmental illnesses and chemical sensitivities. She founded Breakspear Medical Clinic in 1982. Here is one of her books:

- *"Chemical Children: How to Protect Your Family from Harmful Pollutants"* 1987

Dr. Monro, in addition to treating patients at Breakspear Medical, gives global lectures, supervises the training of nutrition students, and contributes to medical articles for various magazines. She has published several research articles in specialized journals, exploring the clinical, diagnostic, and therapeutic aspects of environmental illnesses, including MCS. These resources are valuable for those seeking to understand and manage multiple chemical sensitivity, offering in-depth medical information and practical advice for improving quality of life.

Yukio Yanagisawa is a Japanese researcher recognized in the field of environmental health. He is a professor at the University of Tokyo and specializes in studying indoor environments and their impacts on human health.

- *"Chemical Sensitivity and Sick Building Syndrome":* A book that explores the relationships between chemical sensitivity and sick building syndrome, highlighting the environmental impacts on human health. Written by experts in medicine, chemistry, and architecture, this book examines chemical sensitivity (CS) through 15 chapters structured as lectures. It covers not only medical explanations but also environmental factors, including chemistry and architectural aspects related to this hypersensitivity.

Yanagisawa focuses primarily on indoor pollutants, air quality, and multiple chemical sensitivity. His research has contributed to significant advancements in understanding the interactions between the built environment and health, particularly by examining how chemical pollutants can trigger hypersensitivity reactions in some individuals.

Pamela Reed Gibson

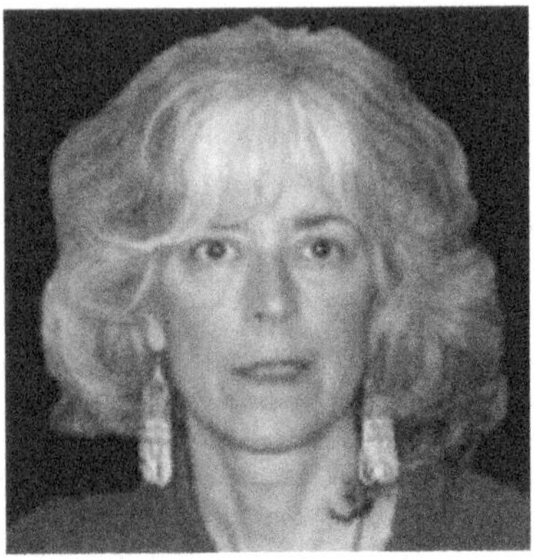

Pamela Reed Gibson is an American psychologist recognized for her research on multiple chemical sensitivity and environmental illnesses. She has studied the psychological and social impact of these conditions on affected individuals. Gibson has highlighted the challenges faced by people with MCS, including social isolation, economic difficulties, and stigmatization. Her work has contributed to a better understanding of patients' experiences and has influenced clinical and support approaches for this population.

References publications

Anne Steinemann

- **Caress SM, Steinemann AC.** Examination of a two-phase population study on multiple chemical sensitivities. *Environmental Health Perspectives*. September 2003; 111(12):1490-7. doi: 10.1289/ehp.5940. PMID: 12948889; PMCID: PMC1241652.

- **Steinemann A.** National prevalence and effects of multiple chemical sensitivities. *Journal of Occupational and Environmental Medicine*. March 2018; 60(3). doi: 10.1097/JOM.0000000000001272. PMID: 29329146; PMCID: PMC5865484.

- **Caress SM, Steinemann AC, Waddick C**. Symptomatology and etiology of multiple chemical sensitivities in the southeastern United States. *Archives of Environmental Health*. September-October 2002; 57(5):429-36. doi: 10.1080/00039890209601433. PMID: 12641185.

Claudia S. Miller

- **Perales RB, Palmer RF, Rincon R, Viramontes JN, Walker T, Jaén CR, Miller CS.** Does improving indoor air quality reduce symptoms associated with chemical intolerance? *Primary Health Care Research & Development*. January 12, 2022; 23. doi: 10.1017/S1463423621000864. PMID: 35019834; PMCID: PMC8822326.

- **Palmer RF, Jaén CR, Perales RB, Rincon R, Forster JN, Miller CS.** Three questions to identify chemically intolerant individuals in clinical and epidemiological populations: The Brief Environmental Exposure and Sensitivity Inventory (BREESI). *PLOS ONE*. September 16, 2020; 15(9). doi: 10.1371/journal.pone.0238296. PMID: 32936802; PMCID: PMC7494077.

Martin L. Pall

- **Pall ML, Anderson JH.** The vanilloid receptor as a putative target for various chemicals in terms of multiple chemical sensitivity. *Archives of Environmental Health*. July 2004; 59(7):363-75. doi: 10.3200/AEOH.59.7.363-375. PMID: 16241041.

- **Pall ML.** Multiple chemical sensitivity as a response to chemicals acting as toxins via excessive NMDA activity. *Journal of Psychosomatic Research*. September 2010; 69(3):327-8; author reply 328-30. doi: 10.1016/j.jpsychores.2010.05.007. Epub June 23, 2010. PMID: 20708456.

- **Pall ML.** Sensitization and stimulation of NMDA by peroxynitrite, nitric oxide, and organic solvents as a mechanism of chemical sensitivity in multiple chemical sensitivities. *FASEB Journal*. September 2002; 16(11):1407-17. doi: 10.1096/fj.01-0861hyp. PMID: 12205032.

- **Pall ML.** The nitric oxide/peroxynitrite theory of multiple chemical sensitivity: central role of N-methyl-D-aspartate receptors in the sensitivity mechanism. *Environmental Health Perspectives*. September 2003; 111(12):1461-4. doi: 10.1289/ehp.5935. PMID: 12948884; PMCID: PMC1241647.

Pamela Reed Gibson

- **Gibson PR, Lindberg A.** Physicians' perceptions and practices regarding patient reports of multiple chemical sensitivity. *ISRN Nursing*. 2011;2011:838930. doi: 10.5402/2011/838930. Epub September 7, 2011. PMID: 22007328; PMCID: PMC3168894.

- **Gibson PR, Sledd LG, McEnroe WH, Vos AP.** Isolation and lack of access in multiple chemical sensitivity: a qualitative study. *Nursing Science Quarterly*. September 2011; 13(3):232-7. doi: 10.1111/j.1442-2018.2011.00606.x. Epub May 20, 2011. PMID: 21595819.

- **Gibson PR.** Out of the world, but not of it: barriers to community access and education for environmentally sensitive individuals. *Women's Health Issues*. January 2010; 31(1):3-16. doi: 10.1080/073993303042823. PMID: 20390633.

- **Gibson PR, Vogel VM.** Illness-related dysfunction in individuals with self-reported multiple chemical sensitivity at four levels of severity. *Journal of Clinical Nursing*. January 2009; 18(1):72-81. doi: 10.1111/j.1365-2702.2008.02439.x. PMID: 19120734.

- **Gibson PR, Placek E, Lane J, Brohimer SO, Lovelace AC.** Disability-induced identity changes in individuals with multiple chemical sensitivity. *Qualitative Health Research*. April 2005; 15(4):502-24. doi: 10.1177/1049732304271960. PMID: 15761095.

- **Gibson PR, Elms AN, Ruding LA.** Perceived treatment effectiveness for conventional and alternative therapies reported by individuals with multiple chemical sensitivity. *Environmental Health*

Perspectives. September 2003; 111(12):1498-504. doi: 10.1289/ehp.5936. PMID: 12948890; PMCID: PMC1241653.

Print on Demand
Legal Deposit: August 2024
ISBN: 978-2-9589939-4-8

National Library of France

Price (including VAT): $17

Made in the USA
Monee, IL
04 November 2026

67383609R00098